IVF DIET COOKBOOK FOR PCOS

Easy and delicious recipes to help you loose weight, improve insulin sensitivity, and boost fertility.

Yvonne J. Schmidt

TABLE OF CONTENTS

INTRODUCTION

When I embarked on the journey that led to this cookbook, I wasn't a nutrition expert or a chef. I was just someone like you, searching for answers, and trying to find a way to overcome the challenges of Polycystic Ovary Syndrome (PCOS) that were standing in the way of my dreams of motherhood.

I vividly remember the frustration and confusion that accompanied my PCOS diagnosis. The doctor's words felt like a heavy verdict. The complexities of PCOS, its impact on my fertility, and the numerous treatment options left me overwhelmed. But deep down, I held onto a glimmer of hope, a belief that there had to be a way forward.

One day, while sifting through countless online forums and medical articles, I stumbled upon a story. It was a story of a woman who, against all odds, managed to conceive and deliver a healthy baby through In Vitro Fertilization (IVF). Her journey was filled with ups and downs, just like mine, but she credited a significant part of her success to the food she ate and the lifestyle choices she made.

That story sparked something within me. It was a ray of hope, a possibility that I could take charge of my

PCOS and fertility journey. And so began my quest to learn more about the relationship between what we eat and our ability to conceive. I devoured every bit of knowledge I could find, tried numerous diets, and explored the world of nutrition.

The result of this journey is what you hold in your hands—a simple, practical, and achievable IVF Diet Cookbook for PCOS. This book is not filled with complicated jargon or fancy words. It's a collection of recipes and guidance based on my personal experiences, my conversations with experts, and my unwavering belief that food can be a powerful ally in the fight against PCOS and on the path to IVF success.

I would love you to join me on this journey. Together, we will explore the wonders of nourishing our bodies, making mindful choices, and embracing the potential of every meal to bring us closer to our dreams. If you've ever felt lost or overwhelmed by PCOS and IVF, I want you to know that you're not alone, and there is hope. The journey might be challenging, but it's also incredibly rewarding.

Now, as you turn the page and dive into the heart of this cookbook, I encourage you to open your mind and heart to the possibilities that lie ahead. Embrace the simple, everyday choices that can have a profound impact on your health and your dream of becoming a parent.

Let's embark on this path together. Your journey starts here. Don't wait another moment—take action, and let's make your dream a reality.
To your health, happiness, and the path to parenthood.

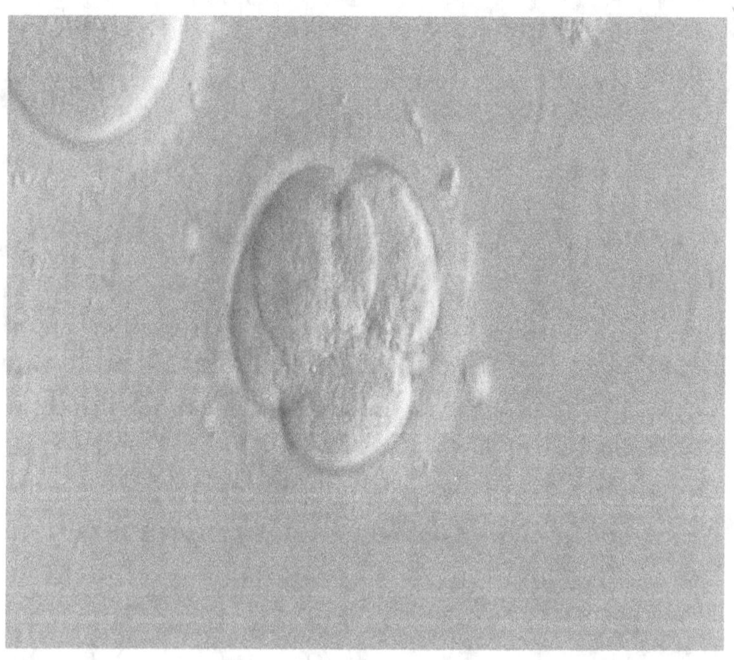

CHAPTER ONE:
PCOS AND FERTILITY

Polycystic Ovary Syndrome (PCOS) can significantly influence fertility, creating a nuanced landscape for those navigating family planning. In this chapter, we'll unravel the essentials in clear terms.

Understanding PCOS: PCOS is a hormonal disorder affecting individuals with ovaries. Common symptoms include irregular periods, heightened androgen levels, and cysts on the ovaries. While not a direct cause of infertility, PCOS can make conception more challenging.

Impact on Fertility: PCOS often disrupts the regularity of menstrual cycles, affecting ovulation. This irregularity can complicate the timing of conception. Additionally, insulin resistance linked to PCOS may contribute to fertility issues.

Practical Tips:
Go for a well-balanced diet that is high in whole foods. Manage carbohydrate intake to address insulin resistance, a common feature in PCOS.

Regular Exercise: Incorporate regular physical activity. Exercise can aid in weight management, improve insulin sensitivity, and promote overall well-being.
Menstrual Cycle Tracking: Monitor your menstrual cycle. Understanding your cycle can enhance the accuracy of

ovulation prediction, optimizing your chances of conception.

Consultation with a Specialist: If fertility challenges persist, seek guidance from a reproductive health specialist. They can tailor interventions to your unique situation.

Control Stress: Excessive stress might make PCOS symptoms worse. Adopt stress-management techniques like mindfulness or yoga.

Partner Communication: Maintain open communication with your partner. Family-building decisions should be a shared journey, fostering mutual support.

Regular Check-ups: Schedule routine check-ups to monitor PCOS symptoms and address any emerging concerns promptly.

Understanding PCOS and its impact on fertility is the first step in a fertility journey. This chapter aims to equip you with practical insights, empowering you to navigate PCOS and fertility with confidence and informed decision-making.

Understanding Polycystic Ovary Syndrome (PCOS)

Polycystic Ovary Syndrome, often abbreviated as PCOS, is a common hormonal disorder that affects many women of reproductive age. But what exactly is PCOS, and why is it important to understand it? Let's break it down.

What is PCOS?

At its core, PCOS is a condition where hormonal imbalances in the body lead to various symptoms and potential health issues. One of the key factors in PCOS is an overproduction of androgens, which are often referred to as "male hormones." These higher levels of androgens can affect the normal functioning of the ovaries.

The Impact on Ovaries

In PCOS, the ovaries might develop small, fluid-filled sacs or cysts, which can sometimes be seen on medical imaging. These cysts are not harmful by themselves, but they can contribute to irregular menstrual cycles and difficulties in getting pregnant.

Common Symptoms

PCOS can manifest in a range of symptoms, which can vary from person to person.

Typical PCOS symptoms and indicators include the following:

A. Irregular menstrual cycles or missed periods

B. Excess hair growth on the face, chest, or other areas (hirsutism)

C. Acne and oily skin

D. Weight gain or difficulty losing weight

E. Hair thinning or male-pattern baldness

F. Skin darkening, particularly around the neck and underarms

The Link to Fertility

One of the significant concerns for many women with PCOS is its impact on fertility. Irregular periods and problems with ovulation can make it challenging to conceive naturally. However, it's essential to remember that PCOS doesn't mean you can't have children—it just means you might need extra support.

Why Understanding PCOS Matters. The first step to manage PCOS is understanding it. The symptoms can be frustrating and even distressing, but knowing what's happening in your body is crucial. By understanding PCOS, you can work with healthcare professionals to develop a plan to address your unique needs and concerns.

A Path Toward Management

In this book, we'll explore how your diet can play a vital role in managing PCOS and improving your fertility. By making informed choices and embracing a diet that supports your body, you can take steps toward a healthier, more balanced life.

PCOS might be a part of your life, but it doesn't define you. It's a condition that can be managed, and this book is here to help you along the way. Let's delve deeper into how the right foods can become your allies in this journey.

Understanding PCOS is the first step towards managing it effectively and making informed decisions to improve your overall well-being and fertility.

PCOS and its Effects on Fertility

Polycystic Ovary Syndrome (PCOS) isn't just about irregular periods and a few extra pimples. It can significantly impact your fertility. Let's explore how PCOS affects your ability to conceive.

Ovulation Challenges

One of the primary ways PCOS affects fertility is by disrupting the ovulation process. A discharged egg from the ovary that is prepared for fertilization is known as ovulation.. In PCOS, hormonal imbalances can lead to irregular or absent ovulation. Without ovulation, it becomes difficult to get pregnant naturally.

Irregular Menstrual Cycles

Women with PCOS often experience irregular menstrual cycles. This means that you might not know when or if you'll ovulate. The unpredictability of your cycle can make timing intercourse to coincide with ovulation a challenging task.

Hormonal Imbalances

PCOS is characterized by higher levels of androgens, sometimes referred to as "male hormones." These imbalances can affect the delicate interplay of hormones required for a successful pregnancy. They can lead to problems with the development and release of eggs, which are essential for fertility.

Insulin Resistance

Many women with PCOS also have insulin resistance, a condition where your body doesn't respond effectively to insulin. Insulin production might increase and blood sugar levels can rise as a result of insulin resistance. This can disrupt your hormonal balance and impact fertility.

Increased Risk of Miscarriage

Unfortunately, PCOS not only makes it harder to get pregnant but also increases the risk of miscarriage once you do conceive. Hormonal imbalances and other factors associated with PCOS can lead to a higher likelihood of pregnancy complications.

The Good News

The impact of PCOS on fertility may seem daunting, but it's important to remember that you're not alone, and there are ways to overcome these challenges. Many women with PCOS go on to have successful pregnancies with the right support and care.

Managing PCOS and Fertility

In the pages that follow, we'll explore how your diet can play a crucial role in managing PCOS and improving your chances of conceiving. By making informed dietary choices and following a fertility-focused meal plan, you can take proactive steps toward your dream of becoming a parent.
PCOS might pose challenges, but it doesn't have to be a roadblock. With the right knowledge and support, you can enhance your fertility and take control of your journey towards parenthood.
Understanding how PCOS affects your fertility is an essential step in taking control of your reproductive health. This knowledge can empower you to make informed choices and explore strategies, like a PCOS-friendly diet, to improve your chances of conceiving.

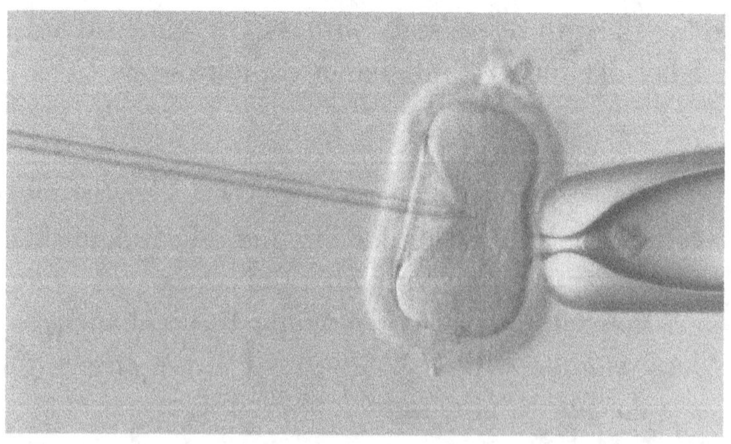

The Importance of Managing PCOS for Successful IVF

For many women with Polycystic Ovary Syndrome (PCOS) who are on the path to parenthood, In Vitro Fertilization (IVF) becomes a hopeful option. IVF can offer a ray of hope when natural conception is challenging due to the effects of PCOS. But why is it so crucial to manage PCOS effectively before embarking on an IVF journey?

Optimizing Your IVF Chances

IVF is a medical procedure that involves fertilizing an egg with sperm outside the body, followed by the transfer of the resulting embryo into the uterus. While IVF is a powerful tool, it's essential to address PCOS before undergoing the procedure to maximize your chances of success.

Regulating Hormonal Imbalances

PCOS is primarily characterized by hormonal imbalances, such as elevated androgens and insulin resistance. These imbalances can disrupt the natural ovulation process and affect the quality of eggs. When you address and manage PCOS through diet and lifestyle changes, you help regulate these hormonal imbalances, creating a more conducive environment for IVF success.

Improving Egg Quality

PCOS can impact the quality of eggs produced by the ovaries. In IVF, the quality of the eggs retrieved is a critical factor in the success of the procedure. Managing PCOS through a balanced and nutrient-rich diet can enhance egg quality, making them more viable for fertilization and embryo development.

Enhancing Ovarian Response

A well-managed PCOS can improve the response of the ovaries to fertility medications used during the IVF process. This means that your body is more likely to produce multiple healthy eggs, increasing the chances of a successful embryo transfer.

Reducing the Risk of Complications

Untreated or poorly managed PCOS during IVF can lead to complications such as ovarian hyperstimulation syndrome (OHSS). By addressing PCOS and achieving better hormonal balance, you can minimize the risk of such complications and ensure a safer IVF experience.

Supporting a Healthy Pregnancy

A successful IVF doesn't end with embryo transfer. It's about achieving a healthy pregnancy and bringing a baby into the world. Managing PCOS before IVF can help create a favorable uterine environment, reducing the risk of complications during pregnancy and childbirth.

Your Journey to Parenthood

In the chapters ahead, we'll delve deeper into how your diet can play a crucial role in managing PCOS and improving your chances of a successful IVF. By making informed dietary choices and following a fertility-focused meal plan, you're taking proactive steps toward a brighter, fertility-filled future.

Remember, PCOS might be a part of your story, but it doesn't have to be the final chapter. With the right knowledge and the power of a well-managed PCOS, you can significantly enhance your chances of a successful IVF and, ultimately, your journey to parenthood.

Managing PCOS is a pivotal step towards achieving success in your IVF journey. By addressing PCOS through diet and lifestyle changes, you're optimizing your body's readiness for IVF, increasing the

likelihood of a successful procedure and a healthy
pregnancy.

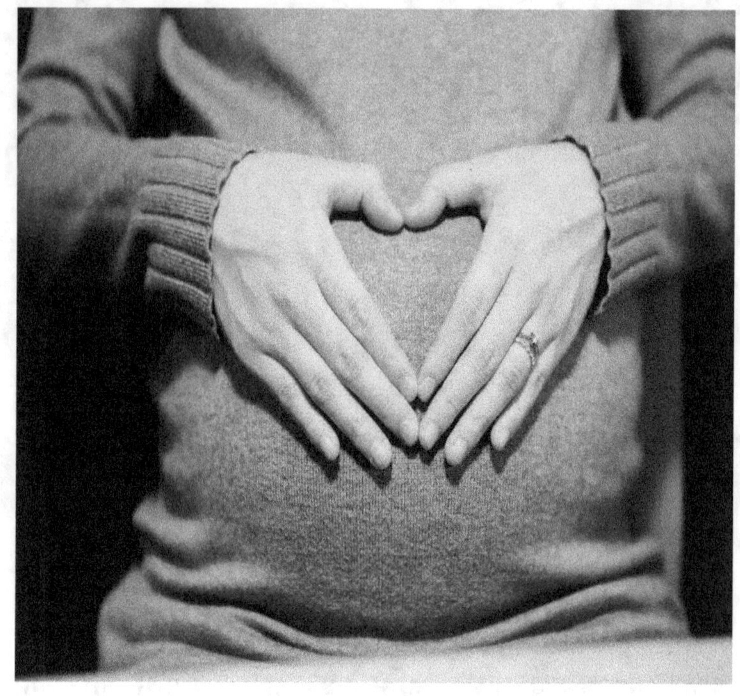

CHAPTER TWO:
NUTRIENT-RICH FOODS FOR PCOS

Navigating PCOS involves making mindful choices, especially when it comes to nutrition. Let's explore practical tips for incorporating nutrient-rich foods into your diet without unnecessary complexity.

Understanding Nutrient-Rich Foods: These are foods dense in essential vitamins, minerals, and antioxidants that support overall health, which is particularly beneficial for managing PCOS.

Practical Tips:
 Bright Fruits and veggies: Arrange a rainbow of vibrant fruits and veggies on your plate. They are rich in antioxidants and fiber, promoting gut health and managing insulin levels.

Lean Proteins: Prioritize lean protein sources like poultry, fish, tofu, or legumes. Protein promotes muscle health and helps control blood sugar levels.

Whole Grains: Opt for whole grains such as quinoa, brown rice, and oats. These complex carbohydrates provide sustained energy and assist in managing insulin resistance. Add sources of healthy fats, such as almonds, avocados, and olive oil. Hormone balance and general health are enhanced by these fats.

Dairy or Dairy Alternatives: Choose low-fat or alternative dairy products rich in calcium. Adequate calcium intake supports bone health.

Hydration: Don't forget water. Staying hydrated is crucial for overall health and can aid in managing weight, a factor linked to PCOS symptoms.

Limit Processed Foods: Minimize processed and sugary foods. These can cause blood sugar spikes and contribute to inflammation.

Mindful Eating: Practice mindful eating. Be aware of portion sizes and pay attention to hunger and fullness cues.

Herbs and Spices: Experiment with herbs and spices like cinnamon and turmeric. They not only add flavor but also offer potential benefits in managing PCOS symptoms. Meal Planning: Arrange your meals so that you get the right amount of nutrients in each bite. Preparation can help you make consistent and wholesome food choices.

Remember, there's no one-size-fits-all approach. Tailor your choices to your preferences and lifestyle. By focusing on nutrient-rich foods, you're not just managing PCOS but also cultivating a foundation for long-term well-being. This chapter aims to simplify your nutritional journey, making it an accessible and effective part of your PCOS management strategy.

The Essential Nutrients for PCOS and Fertility:

In our journey to understand PCOS and how it intertwines with our fertility, we arrive at a crucial crossroad - the significance of essential nutrients. These mighty components that our bodies crave play a pivotal role in managing Polycystic Ovary Syndrome (PCOS) and enhancing our chances of conceiving.

I've been on this path, wrestling with PCOS, facing the highs and lows, the moments of despair, and the glimmers of hope. Along the way, I've learned that what we eat isn't just about satisfying our taste buds; it's about nourishing our bodies, balancing out hormones, and fueling our dreams of becoming parents.

Let's embark on this journey of discovery, where we unravel the power of essential nutrients. Our aim? To make these nutrients our allies in managing PCOS and boosting our fertility. Together, we'll explore the key players in this nutrient orchestra.

1. Folate (Folic Acid): The Builder of Life

Imagine folate as the architect of new life, the mastermind behind cell division and DNA synthesis. It's the nutrient that dreams are built on. As I ventured deeper into my PCOS journey, I discovered that folate is particularly crucial if you're planning to become pregnant. This unassuming B vitamin can help prevent certain birth defects during early pregnancy, ensuring a strong foundation for your baby's development.

Folate hides in everyday foods like leafy greens, beans, and fortified cereals. It doesn't scream for attention, but its role is paramount. It's a nutrient that whispers its importance but is an absolute powerhouse in the realm of fertility and pregnancy.

2. Omega-3 Fatty Acids: The Inflammation Fighters

In the turbulence of PCOS, inflammation can wreak havoc on your body. That's where omega-3 fatty acids step in as the peacemakers. They have anti-inflammatory properties that can help reduce the fiery inflammation that often accompanies PCOS. In my journey, I noticed that including sources of omega-3s, like fatty fish (salmon, anyone?) and humble walnuts, became an essential part of my diet.

But the magic doesn't stop there. Omega-3s also support hormonal balance, a vital element for fertility. They nudge those hormonal seesaws back into harmony, creating a nurturing environment for pregnancy.

3. Vitamin D: The Sunshine Nutrient

Vitamin D isn't just for strong bones. It's a vital player in the intricate PCOS and fertility puzzle.

While I was researching ways to improve my chances of conception, I uncovered the role of vitamin D in regulating insulin levels and supporting ovarian function. It was then that I realized that this nutrient is as essential as the warm sunshine it often derives from.

Exposure to sunlight is one way to maintain adequate vitamin D levels, but if the sun isn't your constant companion, fortified dairy products can lend a helping hand. This nutrient is like a conductor, orchestrating the harmony of your hormonal symphony.

4. Inositol: The Blood Sugar Whisperer

Inositol may not be a household name, but in the world of PCOS, it's a revered figure. I stumbled upon this natural compound during my quest to manage insulin resistance, a common companion of PCOS. Inositol is like a whisperer, gently coaxing insulin sensitivity back to life.

You can find inositol in some foods, but sometimes, especially for therapeutic purposes, supplements might be recommended. For me, inositol became a secret weapon in my journey, helping to stabilize blood sugar levels and opening a door to better fertility prospects.

5. Zinc: The Hormone Regulator

Zinc, a humble mineral, may not be as famous as some other nutrients, but it's a linchpin in hormonal regulation. As I navigated my PCOS challenges, I discovered that zinc plays a role in maintaining healthy menstrual cycles and supporting overall reproductive health.

Lean meats, nuts, and seeds became my go-to sources of zinc, adding a sprinkle of this nutrient to my daily life. It's like a conductor, ensuring that hormonal orchestration remains harmonious.

These essential nutrients are the backbone of your PCOS and fertility journey. They're the unsung heroes, quietly working their magic to support your body's unique needs. By incorporating them into your diet, you're arming yourself with powerful tools to manage PCOS and increase your chances of conceiving.

In the upcoming chapters, we'll delve deeper into the world of nutrients, exploring more key players in this intricate game of nourishing your body for fertility. Together, we'll create a symphony of balanced, PCOS-friendly meals that set the stage for your journey towards wellness and improved fertility.

Remember, your nutritional path is as unique as your fingerprint. It's vital to consult with healthcare professionals or registered dietitians to design a dietary plan tailored to your individual requirements. In the journey of PCOS and fertility, one size does not fit all, but knowledge is the compass that can guide you forward.

In this chapter, we've delved into the importance of essential nutrients in managing PCOS and enhancing fertility. Through personal experiences and descriptive examples, we've uncovered how these nutrients can be the key to a healthier and more fertile you. The journey continues as we explore more of these essential nutrients in the upcoming chapters.

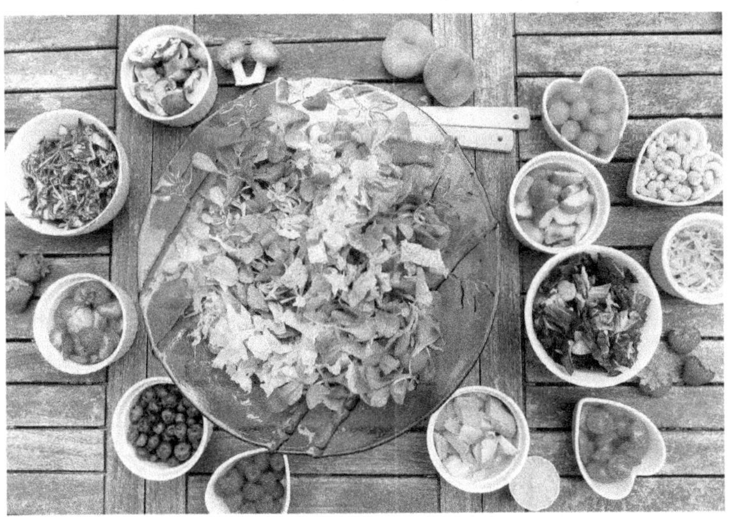

Foods Rich in Antioxidants, Vitamins, and Minerals

In the quest to manage PCOS and enhance fertility, our exploration of essential nutrients continues. Now, let's set our sights on another group of nutritional heroes - foods rich in antioxidants, vitamins, and minerals. These components are like the guardians of our well-being, fighting off the challenges of PCOS and nurturing our fertility dreams.

Antioxidants: The Body's Shield Antioxidants are like nature's shield against free radicals, the unruly molecules that can cause damage to our cells and DNA. PCOS often comes with heightened oxidative stress, which is where antioxidants come to the rescue.

Berries: Blueberries, strawberries, and raspberries are antioxidant powerhouses. They are like a colorful army, ready to neutralize those harmful free radicals in your body. Citrus Fruits: Rich in vitamin C, a powerful antioxidant, oranges, lemons, and grapefruits. They're like your daily dose of sunshine, protecting your cells from oxidative damage.

Nuts: Almonds, walnuts, and pecans are rich in vitamin E, another antioxidant warrior. Think of

them as the bodyguards of your cells, defending against.
damage. Dark Chocolate: Yes, you read that right! When consumed in moderation, dark chocolate can be a pleasant source of antioxidants. It's like a sweet treat with protective powers.

Vitamins: The Body's Allies Vitamins are essential for maintaining good health, especially when you're dealing with PCOS. They aid in hormone regulation and overall well-being.

Vitamin A: Found in sweet potatoes and carrots, vitamin A supports a healthy menstrual cycle and ovulation.

Vitamin B: B-vitamins like B6, B12, and folic acid are vital for hormone balance and are found in a variety of foods, including leafy greens and lean meats.

Vitamin E: Nuts and seeds offer a generous supply of vitamin E, which contributes to reproductive health and the overall well-being of your cells.
Minerals: The Body's Building Blocks
Minerals play a foundational role in our bodies. They're the building blocks for everything from strong bones to balanced hormones.

Calcium: Dairy products and leafy greens provide calcium, ensuring your bones stay strong and your muscle function remains smooth.

Magnesium: Magnesium, abundant in nuts and dark leafy greens, is a vital mineral that helps regulate insulin sensitivity and overall metabolic function.

Zinc: Lean meats, nuts, and seeds are zinc-rich foods that play a role in maintaining healthy menstrual cycles and overall reproductive health.
By including these foods rich in antioxidants, vitamins, and minerals in your diet, you're giving your body a boost in its battle against PCOS and a solid foundation for fertility. These nutrients are your steadfast allies, working tirelessly behind the scenes to support your journey.

In the chapters ahead, we'll dive deeper into the treasure trove of nutrient-rich foods that can nourish your body, regulate your hormones, and empower your fertility dreams. It's a journey where every meal can become a stepping stone toward your path to wellness and improved fertility.
Remember, it's not about a complete overhaul of your diet. It's about making informed choices and incorporating these nutrient-rich foods in a way that suits your tastes and lifestyle. Each step you take

brings you closer to your goal - a healthier, more fertile you.

The Power of Variety: Eating the Rainbow

Incorporating a wide variety of fruits and vegetables into your diet is like painting your plate with an array of colors. Different phytonutrients, vitamins, and minerals are represented by each colour. It's a true testament to the phrase "eating the rainbow."

Reds: Think of tomatoes and red peppers. They're rich in lycopene, an antioxidant that can benefit reproductive health.
Oranges and Yellows: Carrots, sweet potatoes, and oranges are loaded with vitamin C and beta-carotene, supporting your immune system and reproductive health.

Greens: Leafy greens like spinach and kale provide folate and other essential nutrients crucial for fertility and hormone balance.

Blues and Purples: Berries, like blueberries and blackberries, are bursting with antioxidants and vitamins that protect your cells.

Browns and Whites: Whole grains, nuts, and seeds offer a range of minerals, including magnesium and zinc, essential for overall well-being and hormone regulation.

Remember, your journey to wellness and improved fertility isn't just about the individual nutrients; it's about the symphony they create when combined. In the chapters ahead, we'll craft recipes that celebrate the colors, flavors, and nutrient-rich diversity of these foods. Every meal you prepare will be a step closer to your dream of a healthier, more fertile you. As we continue our journey through the world of nutrition and its role in PCOS and fertility, the possibilities are as endless as the array of foods available to us. Your path to wellness and fertility begins with each mindful choice, each bite, and each plate filled with the nutrients your body needs to thrive.

In this chapter, we've explored the power of antioxidants, vitamins, and minerals, and how these essential components can support your journey to manage PCOS and boost fertility. Through clear language and descriptive examples, we've unveiled the nutritional allies in your quest for wellness. The journey continues in the upcoming chapters, where we'll dive deeper into the world of nutrient-rich foods and crafting fertility-focused meals.

Creating a Balanced and Fertility-Friendly Diet

Now that we've met the essential nutrients, it's time to weave them into a culinary tapestry that supports your PCOS management and fertility aspirations. Welcome to the art of creating a balanced and fertility-friendly diet, where the ingredients you choose can be the brush strokes on your canvas, painting a picture of health and hope.

The Harmony of Balance

Balance is the essence of a fertility-friendly diet. With PCOS, your hormonal seesaw may be in disarray. But the food you put on your plate can help restore equilibrium.

The Three Pillars of Balance:

1. Carbohydrates: Carbs are not the enemy. But the type of carbs matters. Choose the complex carbs that are present in veggies, legumes, and whole grains. These are gentle on your blood sugar, preventing spikes and crashes that can disrupt your hormones.

2. Protein: Protein is the building block of hormones and a crucial part of your fertility journey. Lean meats, poultry, fish, tofu, and legumes can provide the protein your body needs.

3. Healthy Fats: Fats play a role in hormone production. Incorporate sources of healthy fats, like avocados, nuts, and olive oil, into your meals.

Eating the Rainbow: The Key to Nutrient Diversity
Remember the power of variety. Eating a wide range of fruits and vegetables ensures you're receiving a diverse array of nutrients. As we've discussed, each color represents different phytonutrients, vitamins, and minerals. These compounds work together in harmony, creating a symphony of support for your health and fertility.

Portion Control: Finding the Sweet Spot Portion control is like the conductor of the balanced diet orchestra. It ensures that you're consuming the right amount of each food group. Eating in moderation helps maintain a healthy weight and balance your blood sugar levels, both of which are pivotal in PCOS management and fertility enhancement.

The Fertility-Friendly Plate

Imagine your plate as a canvas, ready to be painted with the vibrant colors of nutrient-rich foods. Here's a glimpse of what a fertility-friendly plate might look like:

1. Fifty Percent Fruits and Vegetables:
These form the foundation of your plate. Fill half your plate with a colorful array of fruits and vegetables, embracing the antioxidants and vitamins they offer.

2. Twenty-Five Percent Whole Grains:
Whole grains like quinoa, brown rice, and whole wheat pasta provide fiber and essential nutrients. They stabilize blood sugar and keep you feeling full.

3. Twenty-Five Percent Lean Protein:
The remaining quarter of your plate should be filled with lean protein sources. Consider it as the icing on the cake. Protein supports hormone production and overall health.

4. A Dash of Healthy Fats:
Sprinkle a dash of healthy fats like olive oil or a handful of nuts over your meal. These are like the finishing touches to your culinary masterpiece.

The Importance of Consistency

Consistency is the steady beat of the drum in your fertility-friendly diet. It's not about extreme diets or rigid restrictions; it's about nurturing your body with nutrient-rich foods every day. The consistent intake of essential nutrients and balanced meals creates a nurturing environment for your hormonal well-being.

Hydration: The Unsung Hero

Don't underestimate the power of staying hydrated. Water is like a secret elixir, helping your body function at its best. It's especially important in PCOS management, as it supports digestion and the elimination of waste products.

Conclusion: Nourishing Your Journey

Creating a balanced and fertility-friendly diet is a journey in itself. It's a path towards wellness, enhanced fertility, and a brighter future. Remember that the journey doesn't have to be solitary. You can seek guidance from healthcare professionals or registered dietitians who can tailor a plan that suits your unique needs and aspirations.

As we continue our exploration of PCOS management and fertility support, we'll delve even deeper into the culinary world. In the chapters ahead, we'll unveil a treasure trove of recipes that embody the balance and fertility-friendliness we've discussed. Every meal will be a delicious step forward in your journey towards wellness and improved fertility.

The canvas is yours, and the ingredients are your palette. With each meal, you're painting a portrait of health, hope, and a future filled with the joys of parenthood.

In this chapter, we've uncovered the art of creating a balanced and fertility-friendly diet. With a focus on balance, portion control, and nutrient diversity, we've explored how your meals can be a crucial part of your PCOS management and fertility journey. The adventure continues in the upcoming chapters, where we'll dive into recipes that bring these concepts to life on your plate.

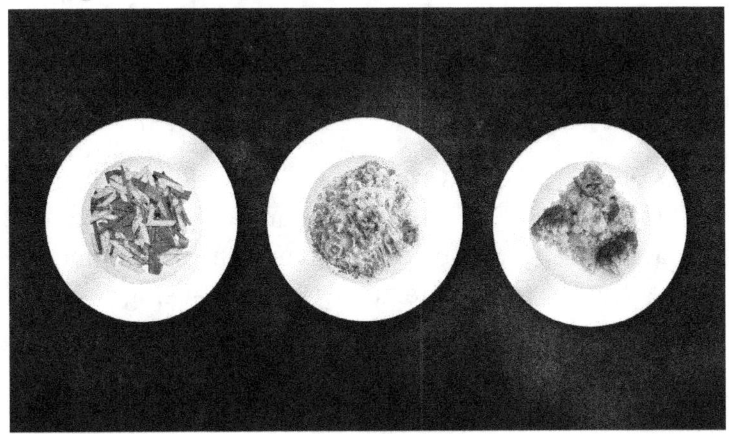

CHAPTER THREE:
PREPARING FOR IVF

Embarking on the IVF journey requires careful preparation and a clear understanding of the process. Let's break down practical tips in a straightforward manner to empower you for this significant step.

Understanding the IVF Process: In vitro fertilization (IVF) involves fertilizing an egg with sperm outside the body, and then implanting the embryo in the uterus. Here's how you can prepare:

Practical Tips:
Consult with Specialists: Schedule a thorough consultation with fertility specialists. Understand the IVF process, potential challenges, and realistic expectations.
Health Assessment: Ensure both partners undergo a comprehensive health assessment. Addressing any underlying health concerns can enhance the success of IVF.

Lifestyle Adjustments: Consider lifestyle modifications. Eat a well-balanced diet, exercise frequently, and learn stress management techniques. These factors contribute to overall well-being and can positively impact IVF outcomes.

Medication Education: Familiarize yourself with the medications involved in IVF. Understand their purpose, administration, and potential side effects. It's critical that you and your healthcare staff communicate openly.

Financial Planning: IVF can be financially significant. Plan for the costs involved, and explore potential insurance coverage or financial assistance programs.
Emotional Support: Recognize the emotional aspects of IVF. Ask your loved ones for assistance, and if necessary, think about counselling. Emotional well-being is integral to the process.

Create a Support System: Establish a reliable support system. Inform close friends and family about your journey, ensuring you have a network to lean on.
Educational Resources: Educate yourself about the IVF timeline, from initial consultations to potential embryo transfer. Anxiety can be reduced by understanding what to expect at each stage.

Maintain Regular Check-ups: Stay consistent with medical check-ups. Regular monitoring ensures that any adjustments needed during the IVF process are identified promptly.

Plan for Recovery: After the IVF procedure, plan for a period of rest and recovery. Make sure your home provides a cozy and encouraging atmosphere.
This chapter aims to demystify the preparation phase for IVF. By approaching it with knowledge and practical preparations, you enhance your chances of a smoother and more successful IVF journey.

Pre-IVF Dietary Recommendations

The journey toward In Vitro Fertilization (IVF) is a momentous step in the quest to bring life into the world. For those of us navigating the path of PCOS and fertility challenges, it's a journey laden with both hope and uncertainty. As we stand on the precipice of this significant milestone, we find that our dietary choices play a critical role in preparing our bodies for the upcoming IVF procedure. In this chapter, we will embark on a detailed exploration of pre-IVF dietary recommendations, a crucial component in optimizing our chances of a successful outcome.

The Foundations of Pre-IVF Preparation

As someone who has been through this journey, I understand the weight of the moment. The preparations you make leading up to IVF can significantly impact the success of the procedure. The first cornerstone of your dietary approach in the pre-IVF period is the management of blood sugar.

Balancing Blood Sugar: The Insulin Connection

Polycystic Ovary Syndrome (PCOS) often comes hand in hand with insulin resistance. The body's response to insulin is impaired, and this can disrupt the effectiveness of fertility treatments like IVF. To address this, there are several dietary strategies you can employ:

1. Embrace Complex Carbohydrates: Think of complex carbohydrates, like whole grains, legumes, and vegetables, as the gentle, steady fuel for your body. They release energy slowly, preventing those rollercoaster-like blood sugar spikes and crashes.

2. Limit Refined Sugars: Processed and sugary foods are akin to blood sugar rollercoasters. They lead to rapid spikes followed by steep drops. In the pre-IVF phase, it's best to minimize these.

3. Prioritize Fiber: Fiber-rich foods, such as whole grains, fruits, and vegetables, offer a triple benefit. They help with blood sugar control, support digestion, and contribute to your overall well-being.

The Role of Nutrient Density

Nutrient-dense foods are a fundamental part of preparing your body for IVF. These foods are packed with vitamins, minerals, and antioxidants, providing your body with the essentials it needs. They are your allies in this phase of your journey. Here's how you can incorporate nutrient density into your diet:

Fruits and Vegetables: Load your plate with the colors of the rainbow. These foods offer a vast array of essential vitamins and minerals. They are the foundational building blocks for your body's readiness.

Lean Proteins: The proteins found in poultry, fish, tofu, and legumes are like the essential workers in your body's construction project. They provide amino acids necessary for hormone production and overall health.

Healthy Fats: Imagine healthy fats, like those in avocados, nuts, and olive oil, as the lubrication for your hormonal machinery. They contribute to hormonal balance and support your overall well-being.

Supplements: Bridging the Gaps

While a well-balanced diet is essential, supplements can serve as valuable allies in ensuring your body is well-prepared for IVF. These are some common supplements to consider:

1. Folic Acid: This B-vitamin is especially important in the preconception period. It can help prevent certain birth defects during early pregnancy.

2. Omega-3 Fatty Acids: Omega-3s support hormonal balance, which can be particularly beneficial when preparing for IVF.

3. Inositol: Think of inositol as the whisperer that improves insulin sensitivity. It's crucial for managing PCOS and, consequently, fertility.

Hydration: The Unsung Hero

Proper hydration is like the unsung hero in your journey. Water is essential for maintaining overall health, supporting digestion, and aiding in the elimination of waste products from your body. The clearer your body's pathways, the more efficiently it can function.

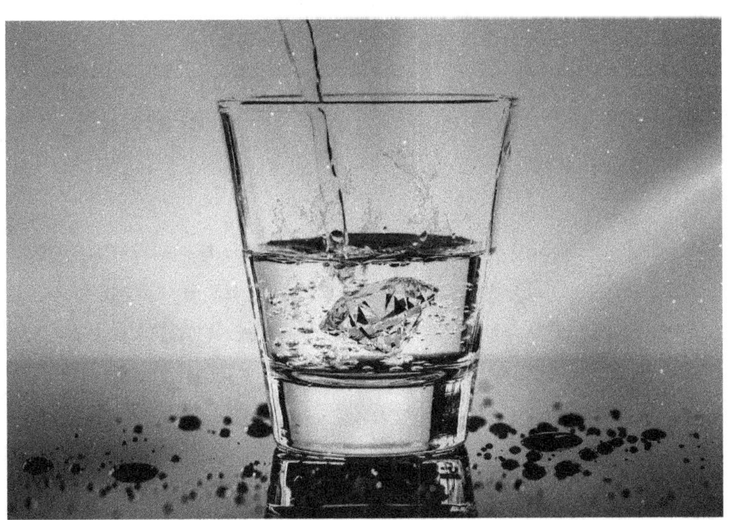

Stress Management: A Holistic Approach

While not directly related to diet, stress management is a pivotal aspect of pre-IVF preparation. The psychological and emotional components of your journey are just as significant as the physical ones. Incorporating stress reduction techniques, such as mindfulness, meditation, or yoga, into your daily routine can be profoundly beneficial.

The Importance of Individualized Guidance

Each person's journey is unique, and their nutritional needs may vary. While these pre-IVF dietary recommendations can serve as a foundation, it's essential to work closely with your healthcare team and a registered dietitian. They can create a personalized dietary plan that caters to your specific needs, addressing any potential nutritional deficiencies and ensuring you're ready for the journey ahead.

As you prepare for IVF, you are embarking on a path that is not only significant but deeply personal. Your commitment to a balanced diet, nutrient-dense foods, proper hydration, and stress management will not only optimize the success of the procedure but also nurture your body for the life-changing journey ahead.

The upcoming chapters will delve deeper into post-IVF dietary considerations, navigating the challenges and joys of pregnancy, and the precious moments of bringing new life into the world. Each page turned brings you closer to your goal – the happiness of welcoming a new life into the world.

In this chapter, we've explored the essential pre-IVF dietary recommendations, emphasizing the importance of balancing blood sugar, nutrient density, supplements, hydration, and stress management. Through personal experience, clear language, and descriptive examples, we've unveiled the nutritional steps to optimize your body for a successful IVF procedure. The journey continues in the upcoming chapters, where we'll dive into post-IVF dietary considerations and the remarkable experience of pregnancy.

Foods to Boost Egg Quality and Sperm Health

The journey to parenthood is a remarkable one, and the health of your eggs and sperm is a critical factor in this journey. While genetics play a significant role, you have the power to influence and improve the quality of your eggs and sperm through your dietary choices. In this chapter, we'll explore practical and straightforward guidance on foods that can boost egg quality and sperm health.

The Impact of Nutrition on Reproductive Health

Nutrition is like fuel for your body. The foods you eat provide the building blocks for the creation of eggs and sperm. What you put on your plate can have a profound impact on the quality and health of these essential components of reproduction.

For Healthy Eggs:

The quality of a woman's eggs is crucial for fertility and the health of the future baby. It's a reflection of her overall health and well-being. Here are some dietary tips to boost egg quality:

1. Antioxidant-Rich Foods: Antioxidants are your allies when it comes to egg quality. They protect your eggs from oxidative stress, which can harm their integrity. Incorporate into your diet items such as leafy greens, berries, and almonds.

2. Omega-3 Fatty Acids: These healthy fats can enhance egg quality. You'll find them in fatty fish like salmon, flaxseeds, and walnuts.

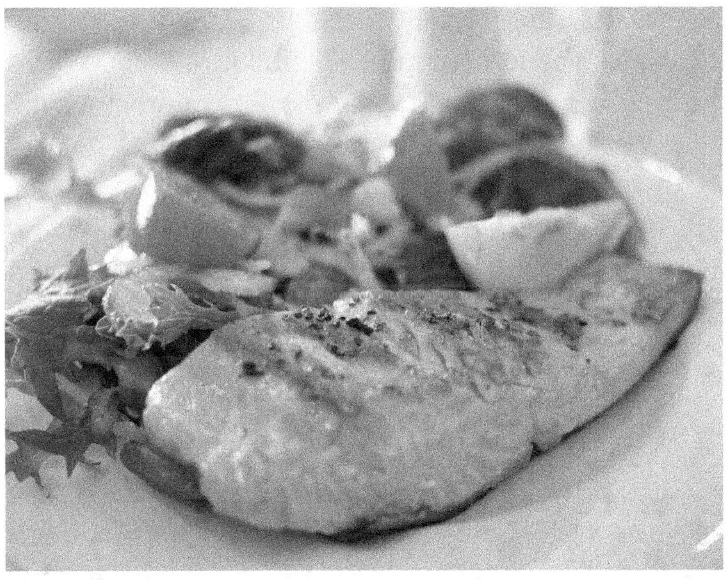

3. Folate: Folate is a B-vitamin that is vital for reproductive health. Leafy greens, lentils, and citrus fruits are excellent sources.

4. Iron: Iron supports the development of healthy eggs. Red meat, spinach, and beans are iron-rich options.

5. Prote it in: Protein is essential for egg quality. Add lean sources to your diet, such as beans, fish, chicken, and tofu.

For Healthy Sperm:

Sperm health is equally crucial for fertility and the health of the future child. The foods you choose can influence sperm quality and motility. Here are some dietary tips for boosting sperm health:

1. Antioxidants: Just as they benefit egg quality, antioxidants are critical for sperm health. Berries, nuts, and vegetables are excellent choices.

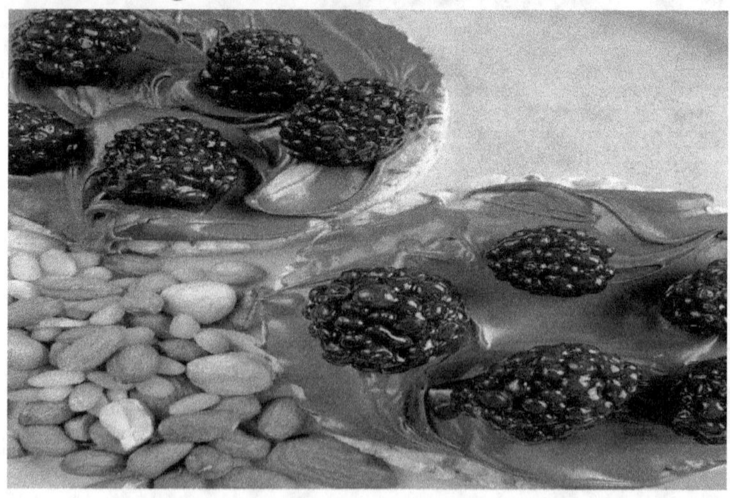

2. Zinc: Zinc is a mineral that supports sperm production. Foods such as meat, oysters, and pumpkin seeds contain it.

3. Vitamin C: Vitamin C has been linked to improved sperm quality. Rich sources include bell peppers, strawberries, and citrus fruits.

4. Folate: Folate is not just essential for women; it's beneficial for men as well. Foods like spinach, asparagus, and beans provide this B-vitamin.

5. Omega-3 Fatty Acids: These healthy fats are known to support sperm health. Incorporate salmon, flaxseeds, and walnuts into your diet.

Tips for Both:

Some dietary choices are beneficial for both egg and sperm health. Here are a few foods that can benefit both partners:

1. Whole Grains: Whole grains like quinoa, brown rice, and whole wheat pasta provide essential nutrients that support reproductive health.

2. Water: Staying hydrated is crucial for reproductive health. Proper hydration ensures the optimal functioning of your body.

3. Leafy Greens: Leafy greens like spinach and kale are rich in essential vitamins and minerals that benefit both egg and sperm health.

4. Nuts: Nuts are a great source of healthy fats and antioxidants. A handful of mixed nuts can be a nutritious snack for both partners.

5. Berries: Berries are packed with antioxidants and are a delicious addition to your diet. They can benefit both egg and sperm health.

Limit or Avoid Harmful Choices:

As important as it is to incorporate beneficial foods, it's equally critical to limit or avoid harmful choices. These include:

1. Excessive Alcohol: Excessive alcohol consumption can harm both egg and sperm quality. When attempting to conceive, cut back on your alcohol consumption.

2. Sugary and Processed Foods: These can lead to inflammation and oxidative stress, affecting reproductive health. Reduce the amount of processed and sugary foods you consume.

3. High Caffeine Intake: High caffeine consumption may negatively impact fertility.

Consider consuming less caffeine by choosing decaffeinated beverages.

4. Smoking and Recreational Drugs: These can have a detrimental effect on reproductive health. Consider receiving help to quit if you or your partner smoke or use recreational drugs.

Consult with a Healthcare Professional:

While diet plays a vital role in reproductive health, it's essential to remember that each person's situation is unique. Before making significant dietary changes, especially if you're dealing with fertility challenges, consider consulting with a healthcare professional or a fertility specialist. They can offer you tailored advice based on your unique requirements.

Conclusion: A Healthier Journey to Parenthood
The quality of your eggs and sperm is a vital aspect of your journey to parenthood. Your dietary choices can significantly influence their health and improve your chances of conceiving a healthy baby. By incorporating antioxidant-rich foods, healthy fats, essential vitamins and minerals, and making beneficial lifestyle choices, you're nurturing your reproductive health.

As you continue on this journey, remember that it's not just about the destination; it's about the path you take to get there. Your commitment to a healthier diet and lifestyle is an investment in your future family's well-being. Each meal you savor, each nutritious choice you make, and each step you take brings you closer to the dream of parenthood.

Your journey to healthier eggs and sperm is a journey of love, hope, and anticipation. It's a journey filled with the promise of new life and the joy of welcoming a precious baby into your family. As you move forward, consider seeking support and guidance from healthcare professionals who can walk beside you on this path.

Remember, you are not alone on this journey, and your determination, combined with the knowledge you've gained, is a powerful force. Your dream of parenthood is within reach, and your commitment to a healthier diet and lifestyle is the key to unlocking that dream. The road ahead may have its twists and turns, but with each stride, you're getting closer to the moment you've been waiting for – the joy of becoming a parent.

Lifestyle Tips for a Successful IVF Cycle

As you approach the pivotal journey of In Vitro Fertilization (IVF), it's not just your dietary choices that matter; your lifestyle plays an equally crucial role. In this chapter, we will explore lifestyle tips that can make a significant difference in the success of your IVF cycle. Drawing from personal experience and evidence-based guidance, we'll navigate the path to a successful IVF journey.

1. Embrace Stress Reduction Techniques:

Stress is an unwelcome companion on the journey to IVF. High levels of stress can affect your hormones, potentially hindering your chances of success. Consider these stress-reduction techniques:

Mindfulness and Meditation: These practices can help you manage stress and anxiety. Dedicate a few minutes each day to quiet reflection or guided meditation.
Yoga: Yoga not only enhances physical flexibility but also promotes emotional well-being. It is a complete way for reducing stress.

Deep Breathing: Simple deep-breathing exercises can help calm your nervous system. Anytime and anywhere can be a good place to practise them.

Therapy and Support: If you're feeling overwhelmed, consider seeking support from a therapist or counselor. Sharing your emotions and concerns with a professional can be immensely helpful.

2. Maintain a Healthy Weight:

Your weight can have a significant impact on the success of your IVF cycle. Both overweight and underweight people may have difficulties. It's essential to strive for a healthy weight range. Consider these strategies:

Balanced Diet: Continue to follow the dietary recommendations outlined earlier in the book. Eating a balanced diet will help you keep your weight in check.

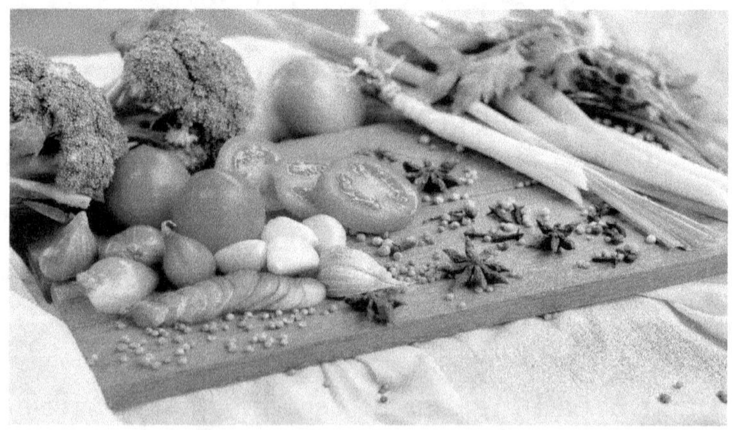

Regular Exercise: Physical activity is crucial. It not only helps you manage your weight but also supports overall well-being. Aim for at least 150 minutes of moderate exercise each week.

Consult Your Healthcare Team: If you have concerns about your weight, discuss them with your healthcare team. They can offer advice, to help you with your particular situation.

3. Prioritize Sleep:

Quality sleep is a silent hero in your IVF journey. During sleep, your body repairs and rejuvenates. Lack of sleep can affect your hormonal balance and overall health. Here's how to improve your sleep:

Create a Routine: Even on the weekends, try to go to bed and wake up at the same time every day. Your sleep can be of higher quality if you follow a regular sleep routine.
Ensure your bedroom is a comfortable place to sleep in order to create a comfortable sleeping environment. It should be dark, quiet, and at a comfortable temperature.

Limit Screen Time: Blue light from screens can cause sleep disturbances. stay away from screens, one hour or more before going to bed.

Manage Stress: Stress might cause you to have sleepless nights. Use the stress-reduction techniques mentioned earlier to help you unwind before sleep.

4. Avoid Harmful Substances:

It's essential to minimize or eliminate harmful substances that can impact your IVF cycle. This includes smoking, recreational drugs, and excessive alcohol consumption. These substances can harm egg and sperm quality, as well as the success of the IVF procedure. Get help to quit using any of these substances if you or your spouse do.

5. Communication and Support:

The IVF journey can be emotionally taxing. Effective communication with your partner is essential. Communicate your thoughts, feelings, and goals to one another. Lean on one another for support. You're in this journey together.

Additionally, consider seeking support from IVF support groups, therapists, or counselors who specialize in fertility issues. These individuals and communities can offer guidance, understanding, and a sense of belonging.

6. Plan and Prepare:

Planning and preparation are key to a successful IVF cycle. Ensure that you have all your appointments scheduled, medications ready, and a clear understanding of the process. Organize your work and personal life to reduce stress during the cycle.

7. Stay Positive:

Maintaining a positive outlook can make a difference. Believe in the process, your healthcare team, and your own strength. Surround yourself with positivity and inspiration. Whether it's reading, music, art, or spending time in nature, find what uplifts your spirits.

8. Be Patient:

IVF is a journey that requires patience. Not every cycle may result in success, and that's perfectly normal. Stay patient, stay persistent, and remember that your journey is uniquely yours.

Conclusion: The Power of Lifestyle Choices

Your lifestyle choices can be a game-changer in the success of your IVF cycle. By embracing stress reduction techniques, maintaining a healthy weight, prioritizing sleep, avoiding harmful substances, fostering communication and support, planning and preparing, staying positive, and practicing patience, you're creating an environment conducive to success.

Your journey to parenthood is a deeply personal one, and the choices you make along the way can make all the difference. The IVF path may have its ups and downs, but your commitment to a healthy lifestyle and a positive mindset will guide you through. As you continue this journey, remember that the future is filled with the promise of new life, love, and the joy of parenthood.

Your lifestyle choices are your contributions to the success of your IVF cycle. They are your commitment to creating a nurturing environment for your future family. With every stress-reduction technique, every healthy choice, every night of restful sleep, and every ounce of patience, you're nurturing the hope of new life and the dream of welcoming a precious baby into your world.

The IVF journey is filled with hope, and your lifestyle choices are the steps that will lead you to that hope's fulfillment. The road ahead may be challenging, but your determination and resilience are your greatest assets. You're not alone on this path, and your journey to parenthood is a testament to your strength and love. With every day, you're drawing closer to the moment you've been dreaming of – the joy of becoming a parent.

CHAPTER FOUR :

MEAL PLANNING AND PREPARATION

Efficient meal planning and preparation are pivotal, especially during significant journeys like IVF. Let's explore practical tips in a simple, straightforward manner to streamline your approach.

Practical Tips:

Make a Weekly Menu: Schedule your meals for the upcoming week. This not only saves time but also ensures a well-balanced and varied diet.

Include Nutrient-Rich Foods: Prioritize nutrient-dense options. A balanced diet should include entire grains, lean proteins, fruits, and vegetables.

Batch Cooking: Prepare larger quantities and divide them into portions. This facilitates quick and convenient meals, especially during busy periods.

Freeze Meal Components: Freeze components like pre-cooked grains, chopped vegetables, or marinated proteins. These can be easily combined to create diverse meals.

Prep Snacks: Have healthy snacks readily available. Pre-cut veggies, portioned nuts, or yogurt cups make for convenient and nutritious choices.

Invest in Time-Saving Tools: Consider kitchen tools that expedite the cooking process. A slow cooker, instant pot, or food processor can be valuable assets.

Label and Date: Clearly label and date your frozen or refrigerated items. This ensures you use them before they lose freshness.

Coordinate with Support: If possible, involve your support system. Whether it's a partner, family member, or friend, shared meal prep can lighten the load.

Variety is Key: Keep meals interesting by incorporating a variety of flavors and cuisines. This adds enjoyment to your meals and helps prevent culinary monotony.

Plan for Treats: While focusing on nutritious meals, allow room for occasional treats. This balanced approach contributes to a positive relationship with food.

By embracing strategic meal planning and preparation, you not only streamline your routine but also prioritize your nutritional needs during significant life events like IVF. This chapter aims to equip you with practical insights for a smoother and more nourishing journey.

How to Create a PCOS-Friendly Meal Plan

Embarking on a PCOS-friendly meal plan is a proactive step toward managing your health and supporting your well-being. In this chapter, we'll break down the essentials of creating a practical and effective meal plan tailored to Polycystic Ovary Syndrome (PCOS). Let's dive into clear, straightforward guidance that empowers you to make informed choices and enjoy a balanced and satisfying diet.

Understanding PCOS Nutritional Needs:

Polycystic Ovary Syndrome (PCOS) involves hormonal imbalances that can impact metabolism and insulin sensitivity. Crafting a meal plan that addresses these aspects is key to managing PCOS effectively. Consider the following foundational principles:

1. Balanced Macronutrients:

Ensure your meals include a balanced mix of macronutrients – proteins, carbohydrates, and fats. This balance helps stabilize blood sugar levels, a crucial factor in managing PCOS. Examples include:

Proteins: Lean meats, poultry, fish, tofu, legumes, and low-fat dairy.

Carbohydrates :Fruits, vegetables, whole grains, and legumes are sources of carbohydrates.

Fats: Avocados, nuts, seeds, and olive oil are excellent source of heart-healthy fats.

2. Fiber-Rich Foods:

Fiber is your ally in managing PCOS. It facilitates satiety, improves digestion, and helps control blood sugar levels., and helps regulate blood sugar levels. Include these fiber-rich choices in your meal plan:

Whole Grains: These are whole wheat, quinoa, brown rice, and oats.

Fruits: Berries, apples, pears, and citrus fruits.

veggies: Brussels sprouts, broccoli, cauliflower, and leafy greens.

Legumes: Beans, lentils, and chickpeas.

3. Mindful Carbohydrate Choices:

Choose complex carbs that have a low glycemic index. These carbohydrates release energy gradually, preventing spikes in blood sugar. Examples include:

Sweet Potatoes: A nutrient-dense, slow-releasing carbohydrate.

Quinoa: A low-glycemic grain high in protein.

Berries: Packed with fiber and antioxidants.

4. Lean Proteins:

Including lean protein sources in your meals supports muscle health, balances blood sugar, and promotes satiety. Consider:

Fish: Omega-3 fatty acid-rich fatty fish such as trout and salmon.

Skinless Poultry: Chicken and turkey breast.

Plant Proteins: Tofu, tempeh, and legumes.

5. Healthy Fats:

Incorporate sources of healthy fats into your meal plan. These fats contribute to hormonal balance and overall well-being. Opt for:

Avocados: Packed with monounsaturated fats and fiber.

Nuts and seeds: walnuts, flaxseeds, chia seeds, and almonds.

Olive Oil: An excellent source of heart-healthy monounsaturated fats.

Practical Tips for Creating Your PCOS-Friendly Meal Plan:

Now that we've outlined the foundational principles, let's delve into practical tips for crafting a PCOS-friendly meal plan that suits your lifestyle:

1. Plan Ahead:

Meal planning is a game-changer. Set aside some time every week to organise your snacks and meals.

 This helps you make mindful choices, save time, and ensures you have the right ingredients on hand.

2. Portion Control:

Manage your calorie consumption by paying attention to portion sizes. This can support weight management, a crucial aspect of PCOS. In order to assist regulate portions, think about utilising smaller plates.

3. Regular Meals and Snacks:

Eat regular, balanced meals and incorporate healthy snacks. This helps maintain stable blood sugar levels and prevents extreme hunger, which can lead to unhealthy food choices.

4. Hydrate Adequately:

Although sometimes disregarded, adequate hydration is essential for good health. Remaining hydrated during the day should be a priority. Infused water and herbal teas can spice up your daily hydration regimen.

5. Experiment with Herbs and Spices:

Enhance the flavor of your meals without relying on excessive salt or sugar. Experiment with herbs and spices like cinnamon, turmeric, basil, and mint to add delicious nuances to your dishes.

6. Listen to Your Body:

Pay attention to your body's hunger and fullness cues. Eat food only when you're hungry and stop when you're full. This mindful approach can help you build a healthy relationship with food.

7. Limit Processed Foods:

Processed foods often contain added sugars and unhealthy fats. Minimize your intake of processed snacks, sweets, and sugary beverages.

8. Include PCOS-Specific Nutrients:

Certain nutrients can be particularly beneficial for managing PCOS. Consider including foods rich in:

Inositol: Found in citrus fruits, beans, and whole grains.

Omega-3 Fatty Acids: Found in flaxseeds, chia seeds, and fatty seafood.

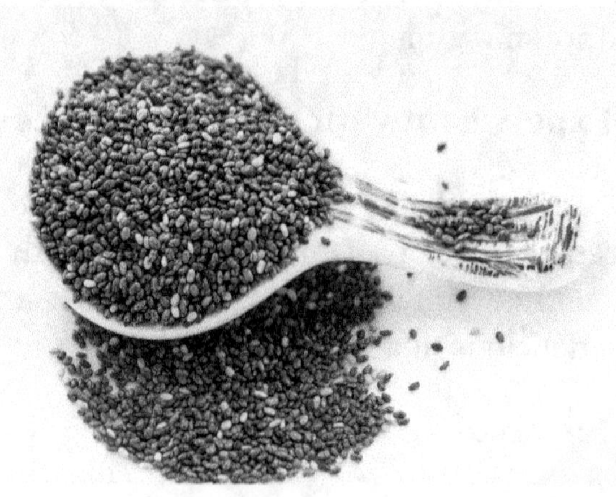

Chromium: Broccoli, healthy grains, and lean meats are good sources of chromium.

Personalizing Your PCOS-Friendly Meal Plan:

Your PCOS-friendly meal plan should be tailored to your individual preferences, lifestyle, and nutritional needs. Consider consulting with a registered dietitian or nutritionist who specializes in PCOS for personalized guidance.

Reflecting on My Journey:

In my own experience, creating a PCOS-friendly meal plan was a transformative step. I discovered the power of nutrient-dense foods, balanced meals, and mindful choices. By incorporating a variety of colorful fruits and vegetables, lean proteins, and healthy fats into my daily meals, I not only managed my PCOS symptoms but also experienced increased energy levels and a greater sense of well-being.

One of the key lessons I learned was the importance of variety. Exploring diverse foods not only kept my meals exciting but also ensured I received a wide range of essential nutrients. From experimenting with different grains like quinoa and bulgur to discovering new recipes that incorporated PCOS-specific nutrients, the journey to creating a PCOS-friendly meal plan became an adventure in self-discovery and nourishment.

Remember, your meal plan is a flexible guide, not a rigid set of rules. Embrace the joy of discovering new flavors, ingredients, and cooking techniques. Your PCOS-friendly meals can be both delicious and supportive of your health goals.

Conclusion: Nourishing Your Well-Being with Every Bite:

Crafting a PCOS-friendly meal plan is a journey toward nourishing your body and supporting your overall well-being. By incorporating balanced macronutrients, fiber-rich foods, mindful carbohydrate choices, lean proteins, and healthy fats, you're laying the foundation for a diet that aligns with the unique needs of PCOS.

Practical tips, such as planning ahead, portion control, regular meals and snacks, and hydration, make the process manageable and enjoyable. Remember, this is a journey of self-discovery, and your meal plan is a tool to empower you in managing PCOS.

As you embark on this culinary adventure, reflect on your personal preferences, savor the joy of creating delicious and nutritious meals, and appreciate the positive impact on your health. Your PCOS-friendly meal plan is not just a menu; it's a celebration of your commitment to well-being, one bite at a time.

Cooking Techniques and Kitchen Essentials

In the journey to a healthier lifestyle, your kitchen is your ally. Understanding essential cooking techniques and having the right tools can turn your PCOS-friendly meal plan into a culinary adventure. In this chapter, we'll explore straightforward cooking techniques and the kitchen essentials that can make your cooking experience enjoyable and efficient.

Essential Cooking Techniques:

1. Sauteing:

Sauteing involves cooking food quickly over medium-high heat with a small amount of oil or fat. It's a versatile technique suitable for vegetables, lean proteins, and even whole grains.

Here's how to sauté effectively:

Use a Non-Stick Pan: A good quality non-stick pan reduces the need for excessive oil.

Cut Ingredients Uniformly: Ensure that ingredients are cut to a uniform size for even cooking.

Avoid Cramming the Pan: Cooking may become uneven if the pan is overcrowded. Cook in batches if necessary.

2. Roasting:

Roasting involves cooking food in the oven at a high temperature, creating a crispy exterior while preserving moisture. This technique is perfect for vegetables, chicken, and certain types of fish. Consider these tips for successful roasting:

Preheat the Oven: Ensure your oven is fully preheated before placing the food inside.

Use Parchment Paper: To prevent sticking and make cleanup easier, line your baking sheet with parchment paper.

Rotate the Pan: Rotate the pan halfway through the cooking time for even browning.

3. Steaming:

Steaming is a gentle cooking method that retains nutrients in food. It's ideal for vegetables, fish, and grains. Here's how to steam effectively:

Use a Steamer Basket: A steamer basket elevates food above boiling water, allowing it to cook through steam.

Time it Right: Be mindful of cooking times to avoid overcooking, especially with vegetables.

4. Grilling:

Grilling imparts a distinct flavor to food and is a healthy cooking method. Whether it's vegetables, lean meats, or even fruit, grilling can add a smoky dimension. Follow these grilling tips:

Preheat the Grill: Ensure the grill is hot before placing food on it for those desirable grill marks.

Oil the Grates: Prevent sticking by oiling the grill grates before cooking.

Use a Meat Thermometer: For meats, use a thermometer to ensure they reach a safe internal temperature.

5. Stir-Frying:

Stir-frying involves cooking small, uniform pieces of food quickly in a hot pan. It's perfect for a quick and nutrient-packed meal. Consider these stir-frying tips:

Prepare Ingredients Ahead: Have all your ingredients chopped and ready to go before you start stir-frying.

High Heat is Key: Ensure your pan is hot before adding ingredients for that signature stir-fry sear.

Stir Constantly: Keep the ingredients moving to prevent sticking and uneven cooking.

Kitchen Essentials:

1. Quality Knives:

Investing in a good set of knives can make your prep work more efficient. A chef's knife, paring knife, and serrated knife cover most kitchen needs. Keep them sharp for safer and more precise cutting.

2. Cutting Boards:

Choose cutting boards made of materials like bamboo or plastic. Have separate boards for different food groups, such as one for vegetables and another for meats, to prevent cross-contamination.

3. Non-Stick Pans:

Non-stick pans are handy for sautéing with minimal oil. Look for quality pans with a durable non-stick coating. They're versatile and easy to clean.

4. Baking Sheets and Pans:

Baking sheets are essential for roasting vegetables, chicken, and more. Invest in quality baking pans for casseroles and baked dishes. Consider non-stick options for easy cleanup.

5. Steamer Basket:

A steamer basket is a simple yet effective tool for steaming vegetables, fish, and dumplings. It's versatile and can fit into different-sized pots.

6. Grill:

Whether it's an outdoor grill or a stovetop grill pan, having a tool for grilling expands your cooking options. Grilling adds a unique flavor to foods without the need for excessive oil.

7. Wok or Stir-Fry Pan:

A wok or stir-fry pan is excellent for quick and flavorful stir-fries. Its design allows for high-heat cooking and even distribution of heat.

8. Baking Dishes:

Invest in various sizes of baking dishes for casseroles, baked vegetables, and desserts. Look for dishes that can transition from oven to table for convenience.

9. Utensils:

Ensure you have a set of utensils, including spatulas, tongs, and ladles, for different cooking techniques. Silicone utensils are gentle on non-stick surfaces.

10. Mixing Bowls:

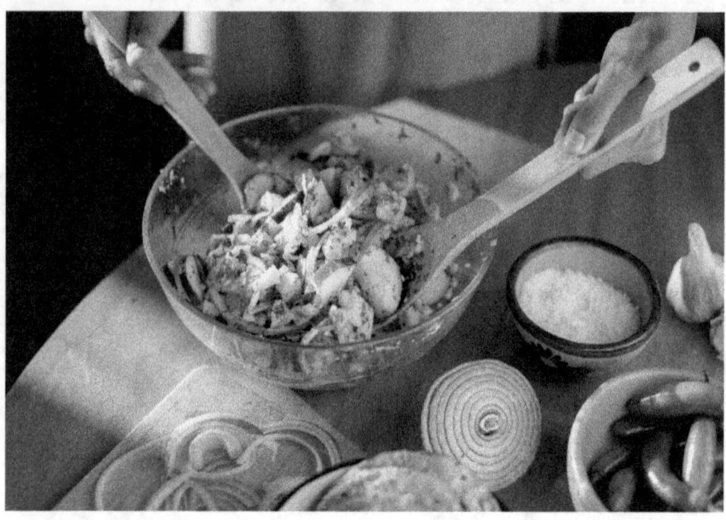

Sturdy mixing bowls in various sizes are essential for prep work, mixing ingredients, and tossing salads. Glass or stainless steel bowls are hygienic and long-lasting.

Organizing Your Kitchen:

An organized kitchen makes cooking more enjoyable and efficient. Consider these tips:

Group Similar Items Together: Store pots, pans, and utensils near the stove for easy access during cooking.

Use Drawer Organizers: Keep utensils and small tools neatly organized in drawers for quick retrieval.

Label Containers: If you store grains, legumes, and spices in containers, label them for easy identification.

Keep Countertops Clear: Clear countertops create a clean and inviting workspace. Store appliances you don't use daily to free up space.

Regularly Declutter: Periodically assess your kitchen tools and utensils. Give away or throw away anything you don't need.

Incorporating Practical Techniques into Everyday Cooking:

Now that you're equipped with essential techniques and kitchen tools, let's discuss how to seamlessly integrate them into your daily cooking routine:

1. Prep in Batches:

On days when you have extra time, consider prepping ingredients in batches. Chop vegetables, marinate proteins, and portion out grains. Store them in the refrigerator for quick and easy assembly during the week.

2. Embrace One-Pan Meals:

One-pan meals minimize cleanup and make cooking simpler. Roast vegetables alongside chicken, or create a stir-fry that incorporates various ingredients in one pan.

3. Plan Meals Around Common Ingredients:

Streamline your grocery shopping and reduce waste by planning meals that share common ingredients. For example, if you buy spinach, use it in a salad, omelet, and stir-fry within the same week.

4. Explore New Recipes:

Keep things exciting in the kitchen by trying new recipes that incorporate different cooking techniques. This not only adds variety to your meals but also expands your culinary skills.

5. Invest in Quality Tools:

Your cooking experience can be significantly improved by using high-quality kitchen tools. While you don't need an extensive collection, investing in a few durable and versatile tools can enhance your efficiency.

Meal Prepping for Convenience and Consistency

In the whirlwind of daily life, meal prepping emerges as a superhero, offering convenience, consistency, and a sense of control over your nutrition. This chapter is your guide to the practical art of meal prepping. We'll navigate the ins and outs, providing straightforward tips to make meal prepping a seamless part of your routine.

Understanding the Power of Meal Prepping:

Meal prepping involves preparing meals or components of meals ahead of time, often in bulk. It's a strategic approach to ensure that healthy, well-balanced options are readily available, even on your busiest days.

The benefits are numerous:

Time Savings: Spend less time cooking during the week by front-loading your efforts on a designated prep day.

Consistent Nutrition: Control your nutritional intake by planning and portioning your meals in advance.

Reduced Stress: Eliminate the daily stress of deciding what to cook by having pre-prepared options at your fingertips.

Cost Efficiency: Buying ingredients in bulk and preparing meals at home can save money compared to frequent restaurant or takeout expenses.

Practical Tips for Successful Meal Prepping:

1. Plan Your Menu:

Select Balanced Recipes: Choose recipes that incorporate a mix of proteins, vegetables, and whole grains for balanced nutrition.

Consider Varieties: Include a variety of flavors and cuisines to keep your meals exciting throughout the week.

2. Make a Detailed Grocery List:

List Ingredients by Category: Organize your grocery list by sections like produce, proteins, grains, etc., to streamline your shopping experience.

Check Your Pantry: Before heading to the store, take stock of what you already have to avoid unnecessary purchases.

3. Invest in Quality Containers:

Choose Reusable Containers: Opt for containers that are durable, microwave-safe, and reusable to minimize waste.

Different Sizes for Versatility: Have containers of various sizes to accommodate different meal components.

4. Designate a Prep Day:

Choose a Consistent Day: Designate a day in your week for meal prepping. It is simpler to create a habit when one is consistent.

Set Aside Dedicated Time: Allocate a specific block of time for meal prepping to stay focused and efficient.

5. Batch Cooking:

Cook Proteins in Bulk: Prepare a large batch of proteins like chicken, tofu, or lentils that can be used in multiple meals. Roast Vegetables Together: Save time by roasting various vegetables simultaneously.

6. Prep Staples:

Chop Vegetables in Advance: Dice onions, bell peppers, and other frequently used vegetables for quicker assembly during the week.

Cook Grains in Batches: Prepare a larger quantity of grains like quinoa or brown rice to use in multiple meals.

7. Layering for Freshness:

Layer Wet and Dry Ingredients: When packing meals with components that should stay separate until consumption (like salads), layer wet ingredients at the bottom to maintain freshness.

8. Mindful Seasoning:

Season Strategically: Avoid over-seasoning if you plan to store meals for several days. Consider adding fresh herbs or dressings just before eating.

9. Label and Date:

Clearly Label Containers: Avoid any mystery meals in the back of your fridge by labeling containers with the contents and date of preparation.

Follow **FIFO**: "First In, First Out" – place newer meals behind older ones to use them in the right order.

10. Freeze Strategically:

Identify Freezer-Friendly Meals: Some meals freeze better than others. Soups, stews, and casseroles are often excellent candidates for freezing.

Use Portion-Sized Containers: Freeze in portions to make thawing and reheating more convenient.

Meal Prepping in Action: A Step-by-Step Guide:

Step 1: Planning

Begin your meal prepping journey with a well-thought-out plan:

1. Review Your Schedule: Consider your week ahead and identify the busiest days when having pre-prepared meals would be most beneficial.

2. Select Your Recipes: Choose recipes that align with your dietary goals and are suitable for prepping in advance.

3. Create Your Grocery List: Based on the selected recipes, compile a detailed grocery list organized by category.

Step 2: Grocery Shopping

With your list in hand, navigate the grocery store efficiently:

1. Stick to Your List: Resist the temptation to impulse-buy. Stick to your list to avoid unnecessary items.

2. Buy in Bulk: When possible, purchase non-perishable items in bulk to save money in the long run.

Step 3: Prep Day

Dedicate your chosen day to the art of meal prepping:

1. Set Up Your Workspace: Clear your kitchen counters and assemble all necessary tools and ingredients.

2. Start with Proteins: Begin by cooking proteins in bulk. This can include baking chicken, grilling tofu, or preparing a large batch of lentils.

3. Simultaneous Cooking: While proteins are cooking, multitask by roasting vegetables and cooking grains on the stove.

4. Chop Fresh Ingredients: Prepare any fresh ingredients that don't require cooking, such as salads or fruit bowls.

5. Portion and Pack: As each component finishes cooking, portion it into your chosen containers. Be mindful of balanced portions for each meal.

6. Label and Date: Clearly label each container with its contents and the date of preparation.

7. Store in the Fridge or Freezer: Depending on the freshness of the ingredients and your planned consumption timeline, store meals in the fridge or freezer.

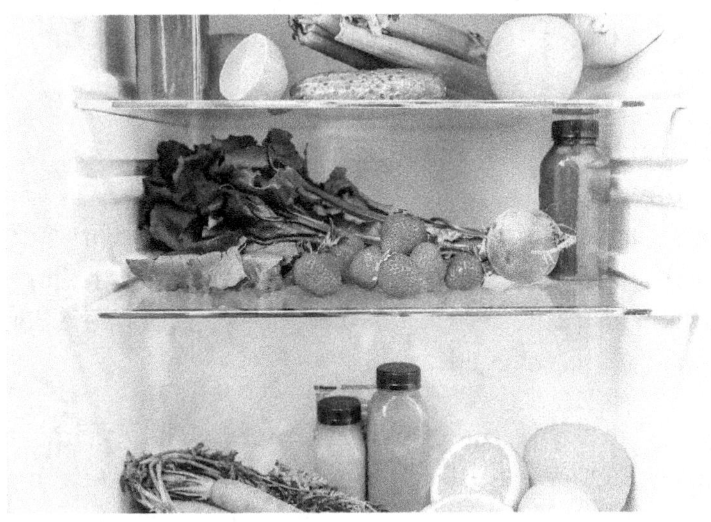

Step 4: Weeklong Enjoyment

Now that your meals are prepped, it's time to savor the benefits throughout the week. Your diligent preparation has set the stage for a week of convenience, health, and delicious satisfaction. Let's dive into how you can make the most of your prepped meals and enjoy a week of stress-free and nourishing eating.

1. Organize Your Weekly Menu: Start your week by organizing your prepped meals into a simple weekly menu. This not only helps you visualize your meals but also assists in planning for variety and nutritional balance. Having a clear overview of your meals can make your week smoother and more enjoyable.

2. Embrace Variety: Variety is not only the spice of life but also the key to a well-balanced diet. As you navigate the week, embrace the diverse flavors and nutrients from your prepped meals. Rotate through different proteins, vegetables, and grains to keep your palate engaged.

3. Time-Saving Convenience: The primary advantage of meal prepping is the time-saving convenience it brings. Whether you're rushing to work, juggling responsibilities, or simply looking for a hassle-free meal, your prepped dishes are ready to go. Enjoy the luxury of a homemade meal without the stress of cooking from scratch every day.

4. Mix and Match Creatively: Flex your culinary creativity by mixing and matching components of your prepped meals. Combine proteins, grains, and veggies in different ways to create new and exciting combinations. This not only adds novelty to your meals but also prevents monotony.

5. Stay Mindful with Portion Control: While convenience is a major benefit, maintaining mindfulness is equally crucial. Keep an eye on portion sizes to align with your dietary goals. Mindful eating ensures you enjoy your meals without overindulging, supporting both your health and satisfaction.

6. Freshness Check: Periodically check the freshness of your prepped ingredients as the week progresses. While many meals remain fresh for several days, certain components may benefit from earlier consumption. Salads, leafy greens, and fruits, for example, are best enjoyed earlier in the week for optimal freshness.

7. Celebrate Flavor Enhancements: Elevate the flavors of your rehcated dishes with simple enhancements. A dash of fresh herbs, a squeeze of lemon, or a sprinkle of your favorite spice blend can transform reheated meals, making them feel like a delightful culinary experience.

8. Freeze Strategically: If you prepared more than you can consume in a week, freeze strategic portions for later enjoyment. This not only minimizes waste but also provides a quick solution for future busy days when you don't have time to prep.

9. Share the Joy: Meal prepping isn't just a personal journey; it's an opportunity to share the joy of wholesome, homemade meals. If you're living with family or housemates, encourage them to explore the prepped options, creating a shared experience of convenience and health.

10. Reflect and Adjust: At the end of the week, take a moment to reflect on your meal prepping experience. Consider what worked well, what you enjoyed most, and any adjustments you might want to make for the upcoming week. This reflective practice ensures that your meal prep routine evolves to suit your evolving preferences and needs.

Conclusion: A Week Well Savored

As you navigate the week with your prepped meals, relish the simplicity, nourishment, and time-saving benefits. A week well savored is not just about the meals themselves but the overall enhancement of your lifestyle. Your dedication to meal prepping has granted you the gift of time and health—cherish it, enjoy it, and look forward to many more weeks of delightful, prepped goodness. Bon appétit!

CHAPTER FIVE:
BREAKFAST RECIPES

Start your day with energy and nourishment through simple yet delightful breakfast recipes. Here are practical tips to make your mornings delicious and nutritious.

Practical Tips:

Overnight Oats: Prepare oats the night before with your choice of milk, fruits, and nuts. An easy-to-eat breakfast awaits you when you wake up.

Smoothie Bowls: Blend your favorite fruits with yogurt or milk and top with granola, seeds, or sliced almonds for a refreshing and filling breakfast.

Avocado Toast: Spread ripe avocado on whole-grain toast and add toppings like cherry tomatoes, a sprinkle of feta, or a drizzle of olive oil for a satisfying meal.

Egg Muffins: Whisk eggs, pour into muffin cups, and add veggies or lean proteins. Bake for a convenient grab-and-go breakfast.

Greek Yogurt Parfait: Layer Greek yogurt with fresh berries, granola, and a touch of honey for a protein-packed and flavorful breakfast. Chia Seed

Pudding: Combine milk and chia seeds, then refrigerate overnight. Top with your favorite fruits or a dollop of nut butter for a nutritious and filling pudding.

Vegetable Omelette: Cook up a quick omelette with veggies like spinach, tomatoes, and bell peppers. Pair it with whole-grain toast for a balanced meal.

Pancakes with a Twist: Opt for whole-grain or almond flour pancakes. Add mashed bananas or blueberries to the batter for added sweetness.

Quinoa Breakfast Bowl: Use quinoa as a base and top it with sliced bananas, nuts, and a drizzle of maple syrup for a hearty breakfast.

Homemade Granola Bars: Prepare a batch of granola bars with oats, nuts, seeds, and dried fruits. These breakfasts are perfect for grabbing on the run. These breakfast recipes are not only delicious but also provide essential nutrients to kickstart your day. Experiment with flavors and find what suits your taste buds and dietary preferences. This chapter aims to make your mornings enjoyable and nutritious with simple yet effective breakfast ideas.

PCOS-Friendly Breakfast Options

Navigating breakfast with PCOS calls for a thoughtful and nourishing approach. In this chapter, we'll explore practical and delicious PCOS-friendly breakfast options. These morning choices aim to provide sustained energy, regulate blood sugar levels, and set a positive tone for the day ahead. Let's dive into a variety of options.

Understanding PCOS Breakfast Needs:

Polycystic Ovary Syndrome (PCOS) often comes with insulin resistance, making breakfast choices crucial for maintaining balanced blood sugar levels throughout the day.

A PCOS-friendly breakfast should focus on:

Balanced Macronutrients: Include a mix of protein, healthy fats, and complex carbohydrates to promote satiety and regulate blood sugar.

Fiber-Rich Foods: Fiber aids digestion and helps control blood sugar levels. Incorporate whole grains, fruits, and vegetables.

Mindful Carbohydrate Choices: Opt for complex carbohydrates with a low glycemic index to prevent rapid spikes in blood sugar.

Protein-Packed Options: Include lean protein sources to support muscle health and provide a steady release of energy.

Healthy Fats: Incorporate sources of healthy fats to support hormonal balance and overall well-being.

Practical PCOS-Friendly Breakfast Options:

1. Greek Yogurt Parfait:

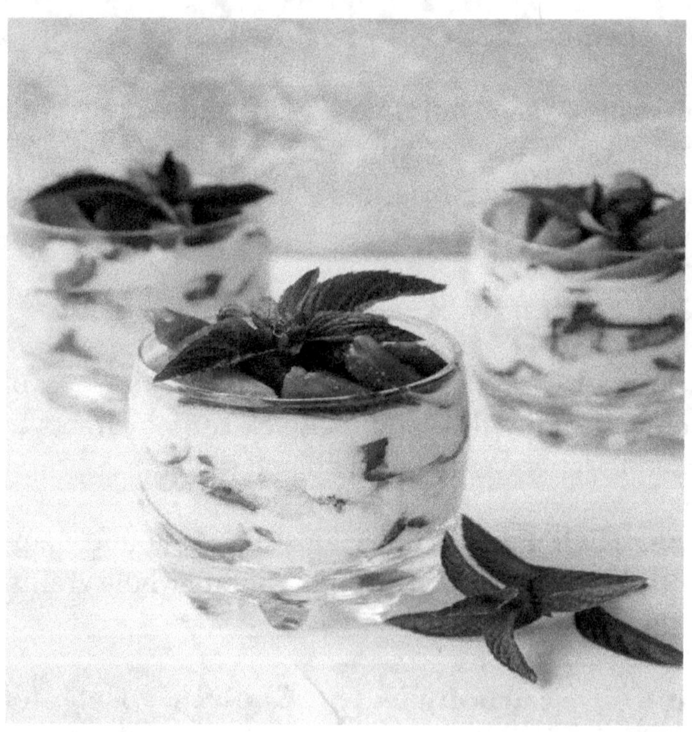

Ingredients:

> ➤ Greek yogurt (unsweetened)
> ➤ Berries (blueberries, strawberries)
> ➤ Chia seeds or flaxseeds
> ➤ Almonds or walnuts (chopped)

Method:

A. Arrange fresh berries and Greek yoghurt in a bowl or glass.
B. To get more fibre and omega-3 fatty acids, sprinkle flaxseeds or chia seeds.
C. Top with chopped almonds or walnuts for a satisfying crunch.

Why it Works:

I. Greek yogurt provides protein.
II. Berries offer antioxidants and fiber.
III. Chia seeds and nuts contribute healthy fats and additional protein.

2. Avocado and Egg Toast:

Ingredients:

> ➤ Whole-grain toast
> ➤ Ripe avocado
> ➤ Poached or fried egg
> ➤ Cherry tomatoes (sliced)
> ➤ Salt and pepper to taste

Method:

A. Spread mashed ripe avocado on toast with whole-grain bread.
B. Add a fried or poached egg on top.
C. Garnish with sliced cherry tomatoes, salt, and pepper.

Why it Works:

I. Whole-grain toast provides complex carbohydrates.
II. Avocado offers healthy fats.
III. Egg contributes protein.

3. Smoothie Bowl:

Ingredients:

➤ Spinach or kale
➤ Frozen berries (strawberries, raspberries, blueberries)
➤ Banana
➤ Almond milk
➤ Toppings: Granola, sliced almonds, chia seeds

Method:

A. Blend spinach or kale with frozen berries, banana, and almond milk.
B. Spoon the smoothie mixture into a bowl.

C. Top with granola, sliced almonds, and chia seeds.

Why it Works:

I. Berries add antioxidants and fiber.
II. Leafy greens contribute nutrients.
III. Toppings offer texture and additional nutrients.

4. Quinoa Breakfast Bowl:

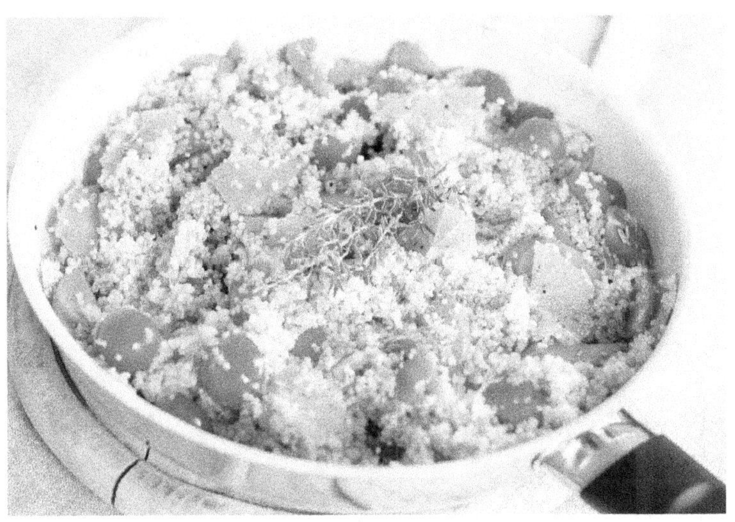

Ingredients:

➢ Cooked quinoa
➢ Greek yogurt (unsweetened)
➢ Sliced peaches or berries

➢ Honey or maple syrup work well for sweetness.

➢ Pumpkin seeds or sunflower seeds

Method:

A. In a bowl, combine cooked quinoa with Greek yogurt.
B. Add sliced berries or peaches on top.
C. Pour honey or maple syrup over it.
D. Incorporate a few pumpkin or sunflower seeds.

Why it Works:

I. Quinoa has a lot of protein and complex carbohydrates.
II. Greek yogurt contributes protein.
III. Fruits provide fibre and natural sweetness.

5. Oatmeal with Nut Butter and Fruit:

Ingredients:

➢ Rolled oats
➢ Almond or peanut butter
➢ Sliced banana or berries
➢ Chopped nuts (walnuts or almonds)
➢ Cinnamon for flavor

Method:

A. Prepare rolled oats according to package instructions.
B. Add a tablespoon of peanut butter or almond butter and stir.
C. Top with sliced banana or berries and chopped nuts.
D. Sprinkle with cinnamon for added flavor.

Why it Works:

I. Oats offer complex carbohydrates and fiber.
II. Nut butter has protein and good fats.
III. Fruits provide extra nutrients and a naturally pleasant taste.

6. Egg and Veggie Scramble:

Ingredients:

➤ Eggs (whisked)
➤ Spinach or kale (chopped)
➤ Bell peppers (diced)
➤ Cherry tomatoes (halved)
➤ Feta cheese (optional)
➤ Olive oil for cooking

Method:

A. In a pan, sauté chopped vegetables in olive oil until softened.
B. Over the veggies, pour whisked eggs and scramble until done.
C. If desired, sprinkle with feta cheese before serving.

Why it Works:

I. Eggs provide protein.
II. Vegetables add fiber and nutrients.
III. Feta cheese offers flavor without excessive saturated fat.

7. Chia Seed Pudding:

Ingredients:

➤ Chia seeds
➤ Almond milk
➤ Vanilla extract
➤ Fresh berries for topping

Method :

A. Mix chia seeds with almond milk and a splash of vanilla extract in a jar or bowl.
B. Once fully mixed, place in the refrigerator and let it thicken for several hours or overnight.
C. Top with fresh berries before serving.

Why it Works:

    I.   Omega-3 fatty acids and fibre can be found in chia seeds.

   II.   Almond milk adds a creamy texture without dairy.

  III.   Berries contribute natural sweetness and antioxidants.

Tips for Success:

→ Prep Ingredients Ahead: Consider chopping fruits and vegetables or prepping certain elements the night before to streamline your morning routine.

→ Mindful Portions: Be mindful of portion sizes to balance your nutritional intake. This is especially important if you're managing your weight as part of your PCOS management.

→ Hydrate: Have a glass of water first thing in the morning. Staying hydrated supports overall well-being and can help control appetite.

→ Experiment with Flavors: Add herbs and spices like cinnamon, nutmeg, or mint to enhance the flavor of your breakfast options without relying on excessive sugars.

→ Rotate Your Choices: Keep things interesting by rotating through different breakfast options. This ensures you get a variety of nutrients and prevents monotony.

→ Listen to Your Body: Pay attention to how your body responds to different breakfast choices. Adjust your meals based on what makes you feel energized and satisfied.

→ Incorporating PCOS-Friendly Breakfasts into Your Routine:

→ Now that you have a toolkit of PCOS-friendly breakfast options, let's discuss how to seamlessly incorporate them into your morning routine:

→ Set a Regular Schedule: Aim to eat breakfast around the same time each day to regulate your metabolism and energy levels.

→ Prepare in Advance: Leverage meal prepping techniques to have components of your breakfasts ready to go. This could include pre-chopped fruits, pre-cooked quinoa, or pre-made smoothie packs.

→ Batch Cooking: Prepare larger quantities of certain breakfast components during your weekly meal prep. For instance, cook a batch of quinoa or sauté a mix of vegetables that you can use throughout the week.

→ Mix and Match: Create variety by mixing and matching components. For example, use the same batch of cooked quinoa in different ways – with Greek yogurt and berries one day, and with sliced peaches and nuts the next.

→ Morning Routine Ritual: Make your breakfast routine a comforting ritual. Whether it's enjoying your meal with a cup of herbal tea or taking a few moments for mindfulness, set a positive tone for the day.

→ Stay Consistent: Consistency is key. While variety is important, having a consistent routine helps stabilize blood sugar levels and supports overall well-being.

→ Plan for Busy Mornings: For days when time is tight, have quick options on hand. This could be a pre-made smoothie, overnight oats prepared the night before, or a grab-and-go option like a Greek yogurt parfait.

→ Remember, your PCOS-friendly breakfast is not just a meal – it's a proactive step toward supporting your health and well-being. With these practical options and tips, you have the tools to create nourishing breakfasts that align with your PCOS management goals.

Nutrient-Packed Smoothies and Breakfast Bowls

Embracing nutrient-packed smoothies and breakfast bowls can be a delightful journey towards a vibrant and healthful start to your day. In this chapter, we'll explore practical and straightforward tips for creating these flavorful and nourishing options. Let's dive into the world of blended goodness and bowlful delights.

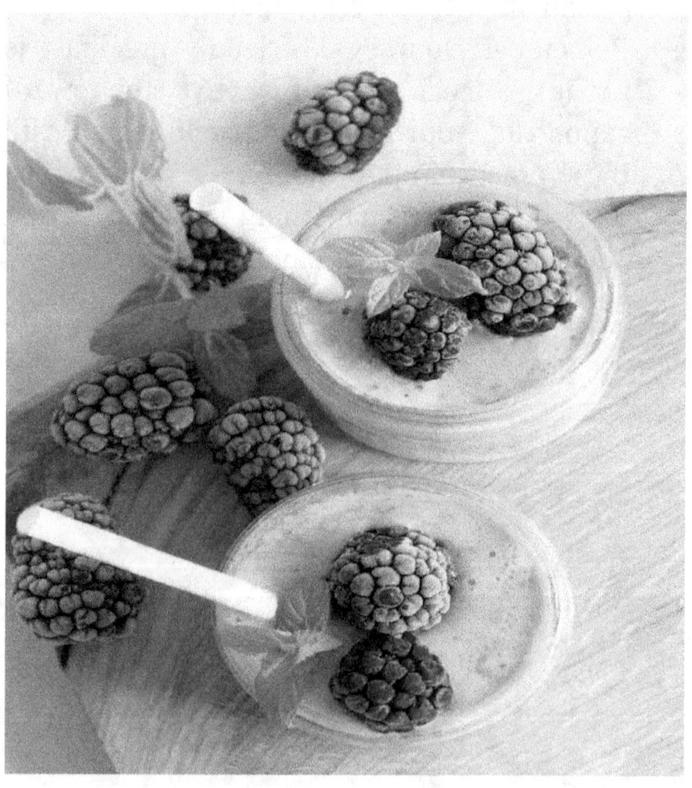

The Art of Nutrient-Packed Smoothies:

Why Smoothies?

Smoothies are a fantastic way to pack a variety of nutrients into one convenient and tasty beverage. They offer endless possibilities for customization while allowing you to incorporate a mix of vitamins, minerals, fiber, and antioxidants. Here's how to craft a nutrient-packed smoothie:

1. Selecting a Base:

Options: Almond milk, coconut milk, yogurt, or a combination.

Tip: Choose a base that aligns with your dietary preferences and provides a creamy texture.

2. Loading Up on Greens:

Options: Spinach, kale, Swiss chard.

Tip: Sneak in leafy greens for added vitamins and minerals without compromising the flavor.

3. Incorporating Fruits:

Options: Berries, banana, mango, pineapple.

Tip: Mix fruits for a balance of natural sweetness and a variety of antioxidants.

4. Adding Protein:

Options: Greek yogurt, protein powder, nut butter.

Tip: Including protein enhances satiety and supports muscle health, especially important for those managing PCOS.

5. Including Healthy Fats:

Options: Avocado, chia seeds, flaxseeds.

Tip: Healthy fats contribute to a creamy texture and help keep you full.

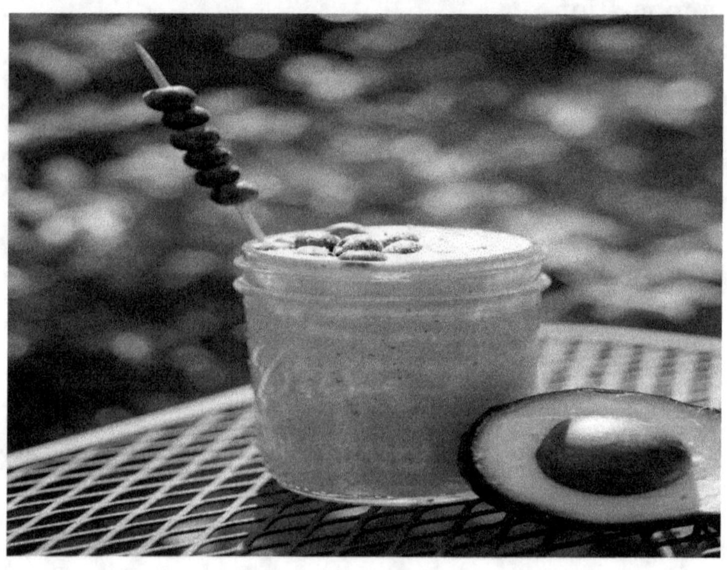

6. Enhancing Flavor:

Options: Fresh herbs (mint), spices (cinnamon), or a splash of vanilla extract.

Tip: Experiment with flavor enhancers to make your smoothie more interesting.

7. Balancing with Liquid:

Options: Water, coconut water, herbal tea.

Tip: Adjust the liquid based on your desired consistency; less liquid for a thicker smoothie, more for a thinner one.

Practical Tips for Crafting Nutrient-Packed Smoothies:

1. Prep Smoothie Packs:

How: On meal prep days, portion out ingredients for multiple smoothies in individual bags or containers. This saves time and ensures consistent portions.

2. Freeze Fresh Ingredients:

How: Freeze fruits like berries and banana slices in advance. This not only adds a refreshing chill to your smoothie but also reduces the need for ice.

3. Balance Sweetness Naturally:

How: Opt for naturally sweet fruits like mango or ripe banana to reduce the need for additional sweeteners.

4. Incorporate Leafy Greens Wisely:

How: Start with milder greens like spinach if you're new to adding leafy greens to your smoothies. Gradually experiment with stronger flavors like kale.

5. Rotate Ingredients for Variety:

How: Switch up your smoothie ingredients regularly to ensure a diverse intake of nutrients. This keeps your taste buds excited and broadens your nutritional profile.

6. Boost with Superfoods:

How: Experiment with nutrient-dense additions like spirulina, chlorella, or acai powder for an extra nutritional punch.

7. Customize for Your Goals:

How: Tailor your smoothie to your specific health goals. If you're focusing on managing PCOS, consider adding ingredients like cinnamon known for its potential blood sugar regulation benefits.

Delicious and Nourishing Breakfast Bowls:

Why Breakfast Bowls?

Breakfast bowls offer a delightful and visually appealing way to savor a variety of nutrients. From acai bowls to savory grain bowls, these customizable creations cater to diverse tastes while ensuring a well-rounded start to your day. Here's how to construct a nutrient-packed breakfast bowl:

1. Choosing a Base:

Options: Quinoa, oats, Greek yogurt, acai puree.

Tip: Select a base that aligns with your nutritional goals and provides a satisfying foundation.

2. Layering with Fruits:

Options: Sliced banana, berries, kiwi.

Tip: Use a mix of colorful fruits to add a variety of vitamins and antioxidants.

3. Incorporating Crunch:

Options: Granola, chopped nuts, seeds.

Tip: The crunch factor not only adds texture but also contributes healthy fats and additional nutrients.

4. Adding Protein:

Options: Nut butter, Greek yogurt, cottage cheese.

Tip: Protein helps keep you full, making it a crucial component for a satisfying breakfast.

5. Including Vegetables:

Options: Shredded carrots, spinach, cherry tomatoes.

Tip: Sneak in veggies for added fiber and micronutrients without compromising taste.

6. Drizzling with Healthy Fats:

Options: Avocado slices, a drizzle of olive oil.

Tip: Healthy fats contribute to satiety and add a richness to your bowl.

7. Garnishing for Flavor:

Options: Fresh herbs (cilantro, mint), a sprinkle of cinnamon, a dash of sea salt.

Tip: Garnishes not only enhance flavor but also add a visual appeal to your breakfast bowl.

Practical Tips for Crafting Nutrient-Packed Breakfast Bowls:

1. Play with Textures:

How: Experiment with contrasting textures in your bowl. Pair creamy yogurt with crunchy granola or add a smooth nut butter to a textured grain base.

2. Mix Sweet and Savory:

How: Don't shy away from incorporating savory elements like cherry tomatoes or avocado into your breakfast bowl. It can be surprisingly delightful to combine sweet and savoury flavours.

3. Use Seasonal Ingredients:

How: Take advantage of seasonal fruits and vegetables to keep your breakfast bowls fresh and exciting. This ensures you're getting a variety of nutrients throughout the year.

4. DIY Toppings Bar:

How: Set up a toppings bar, especially when hosting brunch or catering to different preferences. This allows everyone to customize their bowls to taste.

5. Balance Macronutrients:

How: Ensure a balance of carbohydrates, proteins, and fats in your breakfast bowl for sustained energy and satisfaction.

6. Keep Portion Sizes in Check:

How: While breakfast bowls offer versatility, be mindful of portion sizes to avoid excessive calorie intake.

7. Plan Ahead for Busy Mornings:

How: If mornings are hectic, prepare certain elements of your breakfast bowl in advance. For example, cook quinoa or chop fruits the night before.

Conclusion: Enjoying the Nutrient-Packed Goodness:

As you embark on your journey of nutrient-packed smoothies and breakfast bowls, remember that the key is to relish the process of creating these vibrant and nourishing dishes. Customize them to suit your taste preferences, dietary needs, and health goals.

Recipes for Sustained Energy Throughout the Day

Maintaining steady energy levels is crucial for a productive and vibrant day. In this chapter, we'll explore practical and straightforward recipes designed to provide sustained energy. These dishes incorporate a balance of macronutrients, focus on nutrient-dense ingredients, and are easy to prepare. Let's dive into the world of energizing recipes.

1. Quinoa Salad with Chickpeas and Roasted Vegetables:

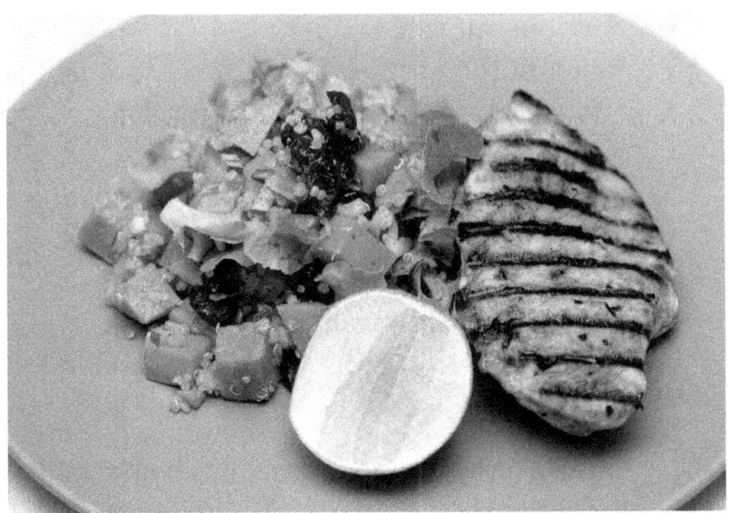

Ingredients:

> ➤ 1 cup quinoa, cooked
> ➤ 1 can chickpeas, drained and rinsed
> ➤ Mixed vegetables (bell peppers, cherry tomatoes, zucchini), chopped
> ➤ Olive oil for roasting
> ➤ Fresh lemon juice
> ➤ Salt and pepper to taste
> ➤ Fresh parsley for garnish

Instructions:

A. Preheat the oven to 400°F (200°C).
B. Toss the chickpeas and mixed vegetables in olive oil, salt, and pepper.
C. Roast in the oven until vegetables are tender and chickpeas are slightly crispy (about 20-25 minutes).
D. In a large bowl, combine the cooked quinoa with the roasted vegetables and chickpeas.
E. Drizzle with fresh lemon juice, toss gently, and garnish with fresh parsley.

Why it Works:

I. Quinoa provides complex carbohydrates and protein.
II. Chickpeas add plant-based protein and fiber.
III. Vegetables that are roasted provide a range of vitamins and minerals.

2. Salmon and Avocado Wrap:

Ingredients:

- ➢ 1 grilled or baked salmon fillet, flaked
- ➢ Whole-grain wrap or tortilla
- ➢ 1/2 avocado, sliced
- ➢ Fresh spinach leaves
- ➢ Greek yogurt sauce (Greek yogurt, lemon juice, dill)
- ➢ Salt and pepper to taste

Instructions:

A. Prepare the Greek yogurt sauce by mixing Greek yogurt with lemon juice and chopped dill.
B. Lay the whole-grain wrap flat and assemble with flaked salmon, sliced avocado, fresh spinach, and a drizzle of the Greek yogurt sauce.
C. Add salt and pepper to taste.
D. Roll up the wrap, slice in half, and secure with toothpicks if needed.

Why it Works:

I. Salmon is a nutrient-rich food that is high in both omega-3 fatty acids and protein.
II. Avocado adds a creamy mouthfeel and good fats.

III. Whole-grain wrap adds complex carbohydrates and fiber.

3. Sweet Potato and Black Bean Bowl:

Ingredients:

> ➤ 1 medium sweet potato, diced
> ➤ one can of rinsed and drained black beans
> ➤ Quinoa or brown rice, cooked
> ➤ Salsa or pico de gallo
> ➤ Guacamole or sliced avocado
> ➤ Fresh cilantro for garnish
> ➤ Lime wedges

Instructions:

A. Roast the diced sweet potato in the oven with a drizzle of olive oil until tender (about 20-25 minutes).
B. In a bowl, assemble cooked quinoa or brown rice, roasted sweet potato, and black beans.
C. Top with salsa or pico de gallo, guacamole or sliced avocado, and fresh cilantro.
D. For an additional taste explosion, serve with lime wedges.

Why it Works:

I. Sweet potatoes are a rich source of complex carbohydrates and fibre.

II.   Fibre and plant-based protein can be found in black beans.

III.   Avocado or guacamole adds healthy fats.

4. Energy-Boosting Smoothie:

Ingredients:

- ➤ 1 cup spinach or kale
- ➤ 1/2 banana, frozen
- ➤ 1/2 cup berries (blueberries, strawberries)
- ➤ 1 tablespoon almond butter
- ➤ 1 cup almond milk
- ➤ Ice cubes (optional)

Instructions:

A. In a blender, combine spinach or kale, frozen banana, berries, almond butter, and almond milk.

B. Blend until smooth, adding ice cubes if desired for a colder consistency.

C. Pour into a glass and start drinking right away.

Why it Works:

I.   Leafy greens provide essential nutrients.

II.   Berries add antioxidants and natural sweetness.

III.   Almond butter contributes healthy fats and protein.

5. Mediterranean Chickpea Salad:

Ingredients:

- ➤ 1 can chickpeas, drained and rinsed
- ➤ Cucumber, diced
- ➤ Cherry tomatoes, halved
- ➤ Red onion, finely chopped
- ➤ Kalamata olives, sliced
- ➤ Feta cheese, crumbled
- ➤ For dressing, use balsamic vinegar and olive oil.
- ➤ Fresh oregano for garnish
- ➤ Salt and pepper to taste

Instructions:

A. Combine the chickpeas, cucumber, red onion, cherry tomatoes, olives, and feta cheese in a big bowl.
B. Pour some balsamic vinegar and olive oil over it.
C. Give the ingredients a gentle toss to ensure even coating.
D. Garnish with fresh oregano, and season with salt and pepper to taste.

Why it Works:

    I.   Chickpeas provide plant-based protein and fiber.

   II.   A wide range of vitamins and minerals can be found in vegetables.

 III.   Feta cheese offers taste and calcium.

Practical Tips for Sustained Energy Recipes:

1. Balanced Meals:

Ensure a balance of carbohydrates, proteins, and fats in each meal for sustained energy and satisfaction.

2. Fiber-Rich Choices:

Choose fiber-rich foods like whole grains, legumes, and vegetables to promote digestive health and avoid energy crashes.

3. Hydration Matters:

Stay hydrated throughout the day. Fatigue and low energy are two things that can be caused by dehydration.

4. Smart Snacking:

To keep blood sugar levels stable in between meals, eat wholesome snacks. Options like nuts, yogurt, or fresh fruit can provide a quick energy boost.

5. Mindful Eating:

Pay attention to portion sizes. Eating mindfully can prevent overeating and promote optimal digestion.

6. Experiment with Flavors:

Add herbs, spices, and citrus flavors to enhance the taste of your meals without relying on excessive salt or sugar.

7. Plan Ahead:

Plan your meals and snacks in advance to avoid relying on convenience foods that may be high in sugar and low in nutritional value.

Conclusion: Fueling Your Day with Energy-Rich Delights

Incorporating these recipes into your daily routine is a delightful and practical way to ensure sustained energy throughout the day. Whether it's a colorful salad, a protein-packed wrap, or a refreshing smoothie, these dishes provide the nutritional foundation for a vibrant and productive lifestyle. Enjoy experimenting with these recipes and tailor them to your taste preferences and dietary needs.

CHAPTER SIX:

LUNCH AND DINNER RECIPES

Simplify your meal planning with these practical and flavorful lunch and dinner recipes. Here's how to create nourishing meals without the fuss.

Practical Tips:

Grilled Chicken Salad: Toss grilled chicken with a variety of fresh vegetables, greens, and your favorite vinaigrette for a satisfying and healthy salad.

Stir-Fry Delight: Stir-fry a mix of colorful vegetables with lean protein (chicken, tofu, or shrimp) and a flavorful sauce. Serve over brown rice or quinoa.

One-Pan Baked Fish: Season fish fillets with herbs and bake with a medley of vegetables on one pan. A fuss-free and nutritious dinner option.

Vegetarian Buddha Bowl: Combine roasted sweet potatoes, quinoa, sautéed greens, and a dollop of hummus for a well-rounded and satisfying vegetarian bowl.

Tomato Basil Pasta: Toss whole-grain pasta with fresh tomatoes, basil, garlic, and a drizzle of olive oil for a simple yet comforting dinner.

Turkey and Veggie Wrap: Fill whole-grain wraps with lean turkey, crisp vegetables, and a spread of hummus or avocado for a quick and portable lunch.

Chickpea Curry: Cook chickpeas in a flavorful curry sauce with tomatoes, onions, and spices. Serve with whole-grain naan or over brown rice.

Quinoa Stuffed Peppers: Mix quinoa with black beans, corn, and spices. Stuff bell peppers and bake for a nutritious and visually appealing meal.

Mushroom and Spinach Quesadilla: Layer mushrooms, spinach, and cheese between whole-grain tortillas. Pan-grill for a tasty and easy lunch option.

Lentil Soup: Simmer lentils with vegetables, broth, and spices for a hearty and nutritious soup. Prepare a large batch for quick, ready-to-heat meals.

These lunch and dinner recipes are designed to be both straightforward and delicious. Feel free to customize them based on your preferences and dietary needs. With these ideas, you can enjoy flavorful and nutritious meals without the complexity.

Nourishing Main Course Options

In the quest for nourishing meals, main courses play a pivotal role in providing essential nutrients and satisfying our hunger. This chapter explores practical and straightforward tips for crafting nourishing main courses. From flavorful protein sources to wholesome plant-based options, we'll delve into a variety of dishes that not only taste delicious but also contribute to your overall well-being. Let's dive into the world of nourishing main courses.

1. Grilled Chicken with Lemon-Herb Quinoa:

Ingredients:

- ➤ Chicken breasts, boneless and skinless
- ➤ Quinoa, uncooked
- ➤ Fresh lemon juice
- ➤ Mixed herbs (rosemary, thyme, oregano)
- ➤ Olive oil
- ➤ Garlic, minced
- ➤ Salt and pepper to taste

Instructions:

A. Marinate chicken breasts in a mixture of fresh lemon juice, minced garlic, chopped herbs, olive oil, salt, and pepper for at least 30 minutes.

B. Grill the chicken until fully cooked, ensuring a golden brown exterior.

C. Cook quinoa according to package instructions, adding a squeeze of lemon juice and a sprinkle of herbs.

D. Serve grilled chicken over a bed of lemon-herb quinoa.

Why it Works:

I. One great source of lean protein is chicken.

II. Quinoa is a unique grain that provides all the essential amino acids for complete protein, as well as complex carbohydrates.

III. Lemon and herbs add flavor without excessive calories.

2. Lentil and Vegetable Stew:

Ingredients:

- Brown lentils, dried
- A medley of chopped vegetables, including carrots, celery, and bell peppers, creates a colorful and nutritious addition to any dish.
- Onion, diced
- Garlic, minced
- Vegetable broth
- Crushed tomatoes

➤ Cumin, coriander, paprika
➤ Olive oil
➤ Fresh parsley for garnish
➤ Salt and pepper to taste

Instructions:

A. Heat olive oil in a pan, then add diced onion and minced garlic. Cook the onion until it becomes transparent and tender.
B. Add the chopped vegetables to the pan and cook until they start to soften, but are still firm.
C. Rinse lentils and add them to the pot along with crushed tomatoes, vegetable broth, and spices.
D. Simmer until lentils are cooked through, and flavors meld.
E. Garnish with fresh parsley before serving.

Why it Works:

I. Lentils provide plant-based protein and fiber.
II. Vegetables offer a spectrum of vitamins and minerals.
III. Spices can enhance the flavor of the dish without the need for excessive amounts of salt.

3. Baked Salmon with Quinoa and Roasted Vegetables:

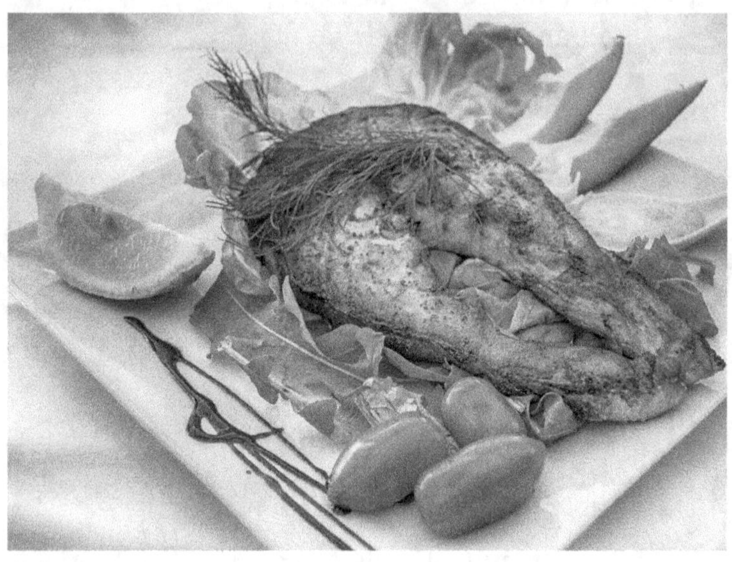

Ingredients:

- ➢ Salmon fillets
- ➢ Quinoa, uncooked
- ➢ Mixed vegetables (broccoli, cherry tomatoes, carrots), chopped
- ➢ Lemon slices
- ➢ Olive oil
- ➢ Dijon mustard
- ➢ Fresh dill for garnish
- ➢ Salt and pepper to taste

Instructions:

    A. Arrange a baking sheet with parchment paper on it and preheat the oven.
    B. Place salmon fillets on the sheet and surround with chopped vegetables.
    C. Drizzle with a mixture of olive oil, Dijon mustard, salt, and pepper.
    D. Bake until salmon is cooked, and vegetables are tender.
    E. Cook quinoa according to package instructions and serve alongside the baked salmon and vegetables.
    F. Add some lemon slices and fresh dill as garnish.

Why it Works:

    I. Omega-3 fatty acids and protein are found in salmon.
    II. Quinoa provides complex carbs and a whole protein.
    III. Vegetables contribute fiber and an array of nutrients.

4. Chickpea and Spinach Curry:

Ingredients:

➢ Canned chickpeas, drained and rinsed
➢ Fresh spinach leaves

- ➤ Onion, finely chopped
- ➤ Garlic, minced
- ➤ Ginger, grated
- ➤ Tomato, diced
- ➤ Coconut milk
- ➤ Curry powder, cumin, turmeric
- ➤ Olive oil
- ➤ Fresh cilantro for garnish
- ➤ Basmati rice, cooked

Instructions:

A. Sauté chopped onion, minced garlic, and grated ginger in olive oil until aromatic.
B. Cook the chopped tomato until it becomes tender.
C. Stir in curry powder, cumin, and turmeric, allowing the spices to bloom.
D. Pour in coconut milk and bring to a simmer.
E. Add chickpeas and fresh spinach, cooking until spinach wilts.
F. Serve over a bed of cooked basmati rice and garnish with fresh cilantro.

Why it Works:

I. Chickpeas provide plant-based protein and fiber.
II. Aside from other vital minerals, spinach adds iron.
III. Coconut milk lends creaminess without dairy.

5. Quinoa-Stuffed Bell Peppers:

Ingredients:

- ➤ Bell peppers, halved
- ➤ Quinoa, cooked
- ➤ Black beans, canned and drained
- ➤ Corn kernels
- ➤ Salsa
- ➤ Cumin, chili powder, garlic powder
- ➤ Shredded cheese (cheddar or Mexican blend)
- ➤ Fresh cilantro for garnish
- ➤ Avocado slices

Instructions:

A. Preheat the oven and prepare bell peppers by cutting them in half.
B. In a bowl, mix cooked quinoa, black beans, corn, salsa, and spices.
C. Stuff the quinoa mixture into each side of a bell pepper.
D. Add some shredded cheese on top, then bake until the cheese melts and the peppers become soft.
E. Garnish with fresh cilantro and serve with avocado slices.

Why it Works:

I. Both complex carbs and full protein are provided by quinoa.
II. Fibre and plant-based protein can be found in black beans.
III. Bell peppers add vitamins and antioxidants.

Practical Tips for Crafting Nourishing Main Courses:

1. Choose Whole Grains:

Opt for whole grains like quinoa, brown rice, or barley to increase the nutritional content of your main courses.

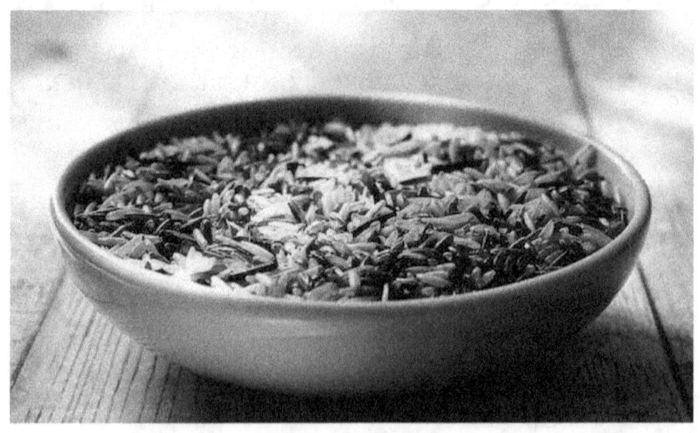

2. Embrace Plant-Based Proteins:

Incorporate plant-based protein sources like lentils, chickpeas, and black beans for variety and a boost of fiber.

3. Prioritize Colorful Vegetables:

Include a variety of colorful vegetables in your main courses to ensure a broad spectrum of nutrients.

4. Lean Protein Choices:

When selecting animal proteins, opt for lean choices like chicken breast, turkey, or fish to minimize saturated fats.

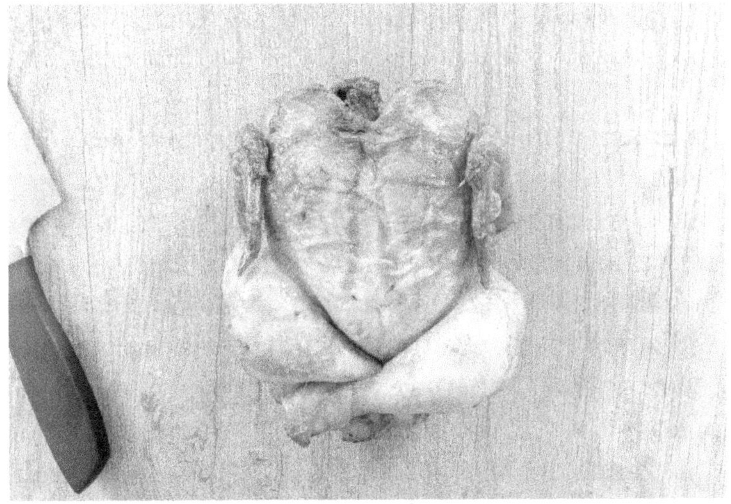

5. Mindful Cooking Methods:

Choose cooking methods like baking, grilling, or steaming to retain the nutritional value of your ingredients.

6. Experiment with Herbs and Spices:

Use herbs and spices liberally to add flavor without relying on excessive salt or unhealthy condiments.

7. Balanced Plate Approach:

Aim for a balanced plate with a combination of proteins, carbohydrates, and fats to support overall nutritional needs.

Conclusion: Crafting Wholesome Main Courses

Nourishing main courses are the cornerstone of a healthy and satisfying meal. By incorporating a variety of nutrient-dense ingredients, you not only create flavorful dishes but also contribute to your overall well-being. Experiment with these recipes and adapt them to your taste preferences and dietary requirements. Whether you're a fan of plant-based options or lean proteins, the key is to enjoy nourishing meals that fuel your body and delight your taste buds.

Delicious and Balanced Lunch and Dinner Recipes

Creating delicious and balanced lunch and dinner options is a rewarding journey toward nourishing your body and satisfying your taste buds. This chapter explores practical and straightforward recipes designed to elevate your meals without complicating the process. From vibrant salads to hearty grain bowls, these recipes aim to strike a balance between flavor, nutrition, and simplicity. Let's dive into the world of mouthwatering lunch and dinner recipes.

1. Mediterranean Quinoa Salad:

Ingredients:

- Quinoa, cooked
- Cherry tomatoes, halved
- Cucumber, diced
- Kalamata olives, sliced
- Red onion, finely chopped
- Feta cheese, crumbledn
- Fresh parsley, chopped
- Olive oil and balsamic vinegar
- Lemon juice
- Salt and pepper to taste

Instructions:

A. In a large bowl, combine cooked quinoa with cherry tomatoes, cucumber, olives, red onion, and feta cheese.
B. Pour balsamic vinegar, lemon juice, and olive oil over.
C. Toss gently to coat all ingredients evenly.
D. Season to taste with salt and pepper and garnish with fresh parsley.

Why it Works:

I. Quinoa provides complete protein and complex carbohydrates.
II. Vegetables offer an array of vitamins and minerals.
III. Feta cheese adds a burst of flavor and a dose of calcium.

2. Teriyaki Salmon Bowl:

Ingredients:

➢ Salmon fillets, grilled or baked
➢ Brown rice, cooked
➢ Broccoli florets, steamed
➢ Carrots, julienned
➢ Edamame, shelled
➢ Teriyaki sauce
➢ Sesame seeds for garnish

> Green onions, sliced

Instructions:

A. Grill or bake salmon fillets until fully cooked.
B. Assemble bowls with a base of cooked brown rice, topped with steamed broccoli, julienned carrots, and edamame.
C. Place grilled or baked salmon on top.
D. Add a teriyaki sauce drizzle and decorate with chopped green onions and sesame seeds.

Why it Works:

I. Salmon is a lean protein with healthy fats.
II. Brown rice offers complex carbohydrates and fiber.
III. Vegetables contribute vitamins and minerals.

3. Chickpea Caesar Salad:

Ingredients:

> Romaine lettuce, chopped
> Chickpeas, roasted or canned
> Cherry tomatoes, halved
> Parmesan cheese, shaved
> Caesar dressing (homemade or store-bought)
> Croutons
> Lemon wedges for garnish
> Salt and pepper to taste

Instructions:

A. In a large bowl, combine chopped romaine lettuce with roasted or canned chickpeas, cherry tomatoes, and shaved Parmesan cheese.
B. Toss to coat evenly with Caesar dressing.
C. Top with croutons and garnish with lemon wedges.
D. Season with salt and pepper to taste.

Why it Works:

I. Chickpeas provide plant-based protein and fiber.
II. Romaine lettuce offers a low-calorie base with vitamins and minerals.
III. Caesar dressing adds creaminess without excess calories.

4. Quinoa-Stuffed Acorn Squash:

Ingredients:

- Acorn squash, halved and seeds removed
- Quinoa, cooked
- Black beans, canned and drained
- Corn kernels
- Red bell pepper, diced
- Cilantro, chopped
- Lime juice

➤ Avocado slices for serving
➤ Salt and pepper to taste

Instructions:

A. Preheat the oven and roast acorn squash halves until tender.
B. In a bowl, mix cooked quinoa, black beans, corn, diced red bell pepper, cilantro, and lime juice.
C. Place the quinoa mixture inside each half of the acorn squash.
D. Serve with avocado slices on top.
E. Season with salt and pepper to taste.

Why it Works:

I. Acorn squash provides vitamins and antioxidants.
II. Quinoa provides complex carbs and a whole protein.
III. Black beans provide fibre and plant-based protein.

5. Stir-Fried Tofu and Vegetable Noodles:

Ingredients:

➤ Tofu, extra firm, cubed
➤ Whole-grain or rice noodles, cooked
➤ Broccoli florets
➤ Bell peppers, thinly sliced

➢ Carrots, julienned
➢ Snow peas, trimmed
➢ Sesame oil and soy sauce for stir-frying
➢ Sesame seeds and green onions for garnish

Instructions:

A. Press tofu to remove excess water, then cube it.
B. Stir-fry tofu until golden brown in sesame oil.
C. Add broccoli, bell peppers, carrots, and snow peas to the pan.
D. Stir in cooked noodles and drizzle with soy sauce.
E. Garnish with sesame seeds and sliced green onions.

Why it Works:

I. Tofu provides plant-based protein.
II. Whole-grain or rice noodles offer complex carbohydrates.
III. Vegetables contribute a variety of nutrients and fiber.
IV. Practical Tips for Crafting Delicious and Balanced Lunch and Dinner Recipes:

1. Mindful Portion Control:

Be mindful of portion sizes to avoid overeating, especially with calorie-dense ingredients like oils or dressings.

2. Prep Ingredients in Advance:

Chop vegetables, marinate proteins, or cook grains in advance for quicker assembly during mealtime.

3. Experiment with Global Flavors:

Explore global cuisines to introduce variety and exciting flavors into your meals. Incorporate spices, herbs, or sauces to add depth.

4. Balance Macronutrients:

Ensure a balance of proteins, carbohydrates, and fats in your meals for sustained energy and satisfaction.

5. Utilize Leftovers Creatively:

Transform leftovers into new meals by combining them with fresh ingredients or using them as components in different dishes.

6. Incorporate Healthy Fats:

Include sources of healthy fats, such as avocados, nuts, or olive oil, to enhance the flavor and promote satiety.

7. Choose Whole and Unprocessed Foods:

Prioritize whole, unprocessed foods to maximize nutritional benefits and minimize unnecessary additives or preservatives.

8. Hydration:

Remember to stay hydrated throughout the day. Adequate water intake supports digestion and overall well-being.

9. Mindful Eating Practices:

Practice mindful eating by savoring each bite, paying attention to hunger and fullness cues, and enjoying the sensory experience of your meals.

10. Flexibility and Adaptation:

Feel free to adapt recipes based on your preferences, dietary needs, or ingredient availability. Cooking should be an enjoyable and flexible experience.

Conclusion: A Culinary Adventure in Balanced Dining

Crafting delicious and balanced lunch and dinner options is an exciting culinary adventure. These recipes offer a blend of flavors, textures, and nutritional benefits to elevate your meals while maintaining simplicity. Whether you're a fan of vibrant salads, hearty bowls, or stir-fried delights, the key is to enjoy the process of creating and savoring nourishing dishes. Experiment with these recipes, make them your own, and embark on a delightful journey toward balanced and satisfying dining experiences.

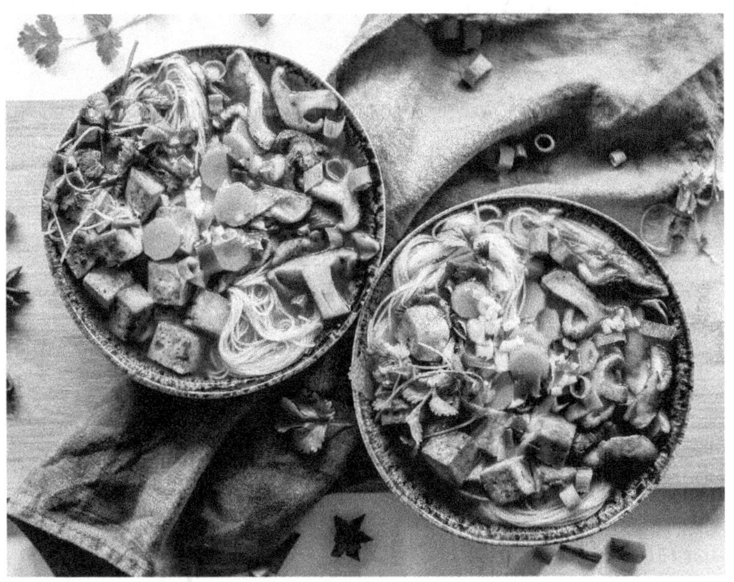

Making Mealtime Enjoyable and Fertility-Focused

Mealtime is more than just nourishment; it's an opportunity to support your fertility journey while savoring the pleasures of food. This chapter explores practical and straightforward tips for making mealtime enjoyable and fertility-focused. From creating a positive eating environment to incorporating fertility-boosting ingredients, these suggestions aim to enhance your overall well-being. Let's embark on this journey.

1. Create a Relaxing Atmosphere:

Set the tone for a pleasant meal by creating a calm and inviting atmosphere. Dim the lights, play soothing music, or light a candle. Taking a moment to unwind before eating can positively impact digestion and enhance the overall dining experience.

2. Mindful Eating Practices:

Engage in mindful eating by paying attention to the sensory aspects of your meal. Take note of your food's flavours, textures, and colours. Chew slowly and savor each bite. Mindful eating promotes better digestion and allows you to appreciate the nourishment you're providing your body.

3. Fertility-Boosting Ingredients:

Incorporate fertility-boosting ingredients into your meals. Foods rich in antioxidants, such as berries, leafy greens, and nuts, can support reproductive health. Omega-3 fatty acids found in fish, flaxseeds, and walnuts may also have positive effects on fertility. Experiment with including these ingredients in various dishes to enhance your fertility-focused approach.

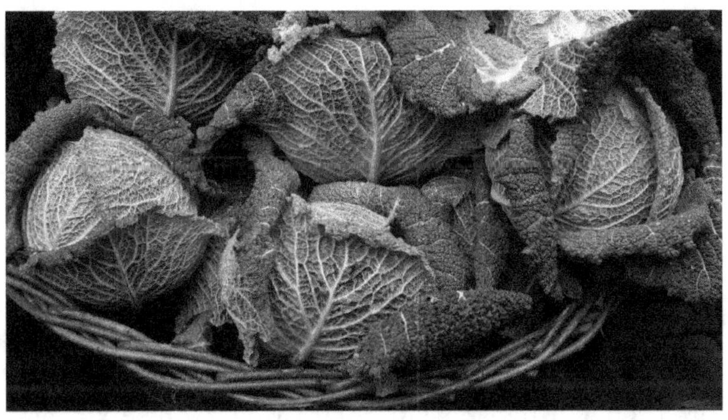

4. Balanced Meals for Hormonal Health:

Design your meals to support hormonal balance. Ensure a balance of macronutrients, including complex carbohydrates, lean proteins, and healthy fats. Whole grains, lean proteins, and avocados are examples of foods that contribute to stable blood sugar levels and hormonal health.

5. Mind-Body Connection:

Cultivate a strong mind-body connection during meals. Use mealtime as an opportunity to relax and connect with your body. Acknowledge the nourishment each bite provides, fostering a positive relationship with food and supporting your overall well-being.

6. Meal Planning for Consistency:

Plan your meals in advance to create consistency in your dietary habits. Having a well-thought-out meal plan reduces stress around mealtimes and ensures you have fertility-friendly options readily available. This approach also allows you to include a variety of nutrient-dense foods throughout the week.

7. Include Folate-Rich Foods:

Folate is a crucial nutrient for fertility and early pregnancy. Incorporate folate-rich foods like leafy greens, lentils, and citrus fruits into your meals. These foods support healthy cell division and can contribute to reproductive well-being.

8. Hydration for Fertility:

Stay adequately hydrated to support fertility. Water plays a vital role in various bodily functions, including reproductive health. Aim to drink enough water throughout the day, and consider incorporating hydrating foods like watermelon, cucumber, and oranges into your meals.

9. Connection Through Cooking:

Involve your partner or loved ones in the cooking process. Cooking together can be a bonding experience and may contribute to a positive and supportive environment. Share the joy of preparing fertility-focused meals and experimenting with new recipes as a team.

10. Mindful Portion Control:

Practice mindful portion control to ensure you're providing your body with the right amount of nutrients. Recognise when you are hungry and full, and steer clear of restricted eating practises. A balanced and moderate approach to portion sizes supports overall well-being.

11. Celebrate Food Diversity:

Embrace a diverse range of foods to ensure you're obtaining a broad spectrum of nutrients. Celebrate the variety of flavors, colors, and textures on your plate. A diverse and colorful diet provides different micronutrients that contribute to overall health and fertility.

12. Positive Affirmations:

Incorporate positive affirmations into your mealtime routine. When you put food on your plate, take a moment to be grateful for what you have. Positive affirmations can create a positive mindset around food and contribute to a supportive fertility-focused approach.

13. Listen to Your Body:

Pay attention to your body's cues both during and after eating. Take note of your feelings after eating various foods. If you notice specific reactions or sensitivities, consider adjusting your diet accordingly. Listening to your body's cues promotes self-awareness and allows for personalized dietary choices.

14. Enjoyable Fertility-Focused Recipes:

Explore and experiment with enjoyable fertility-focused recipes. From nutrient-packed smoothies to colorful salads, there are numerous ways to incorporate fertility-boosting ingredients into your meals. Make the process of nourishing your body an enjoyable and creative experience.

15. Educate Yourself:

Take the time to educate yourself about fertility-friendly foods and their benefits. Understanding the nutritional aspects that support reproductive health empowers you to make informed choices and tailor your meals to your specific needs.

Conclusion: Cultivating Fertility Through Enjoyable Meals

Making mealtime enjoyable and fertility-focused is a holistic approach that combines nourishing your body with the joy of savoring delicious and wholesome foods. By creating a positive eating environment, incorporating fertility-boosting ingredients, and practicing mindful habits, you contribute to your overall well-being and support your fertility journey. Remember that each meal is an opportunity to nourish your body and embrace the pleasure of food. Explore, experiment, and enjoy the process of making mealtime a delightful and fertility-focused experience.

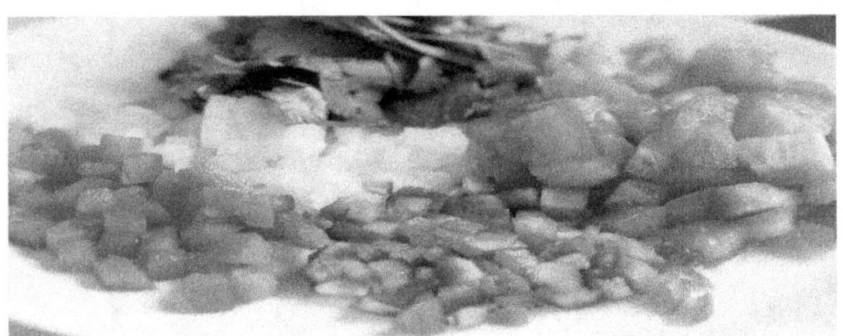

CHAPTER SEVEN:

SNACKS AND SWEETS

Satisfy your cravings with smart and balanced snack options. Here are practical tips for enjoying snacks and sweets in a way that aligns with your PCOS-friendly lifestyle.

Practical Tips:

Nut Butter on Whole-Grain Crackers: Spread almond or peanut butter on whole-grain crackers for a delightful combination of protein and complex carbs. Berries on Top of Greek Yoghurt: Savour a dish of Greek yoghurt garnished with juicy berries. The protein in yogurt keeps you full, and the berries add natural sweetness.

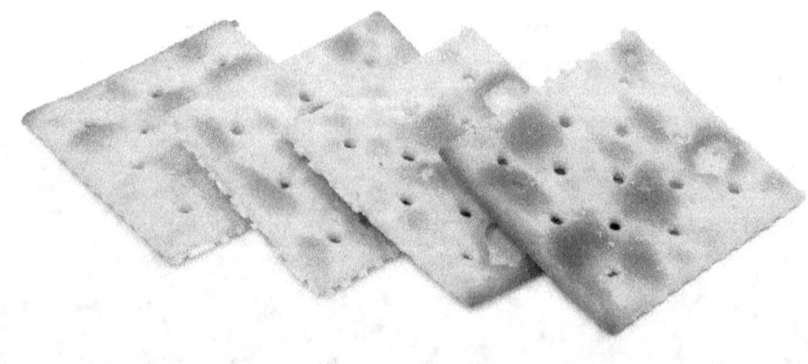

Trail Mix: Create your trail mix with a mix of nuts, seeds, and a touch of dark chocolate. Portion it for convenient and satisfying on-the-go snacks.

Sliced Apple with Cheese: Pair sliced apples with a serving of cheese for a balanced snack that combines fiber, vitamins, and protein.

Roasted Chickpeas: Roast chickpeas with a sprinkle of your favorite spices for a crunchy and protein-packed snack.

Dark Chocolate-Covered Almonds: Indulge in moderation with dark chocolate-covered almonds for a sweet treat that provides antioxidants and healthy fats.

Cottage Cheese with Pineapple: Combine cottage cheese with pineapple chunks for a refreshing and protein-rich snack.

Homemade Popcorn: Make your popcorn and season it with a mix of herbs or nutritional yeast for a flavorful, guilt-free snack.

Chia Seed Pudding with Fruit: Create a chia seed pudding by mixing chia seeds with milk and topping it with your favorite fruits for a satisfying and nutrient-rich sweet option.

Frozen Grapes: Freeze grapes for a naturally sweet and refreshing snack. They're like bite-sized popsicles.

Approach snacks and sweets with a mindful and balanced mindset. These practical ideas offer a blend of flavors and nutrition, enhancing your snacking experience while aligning with your PCOS-friendly goals.

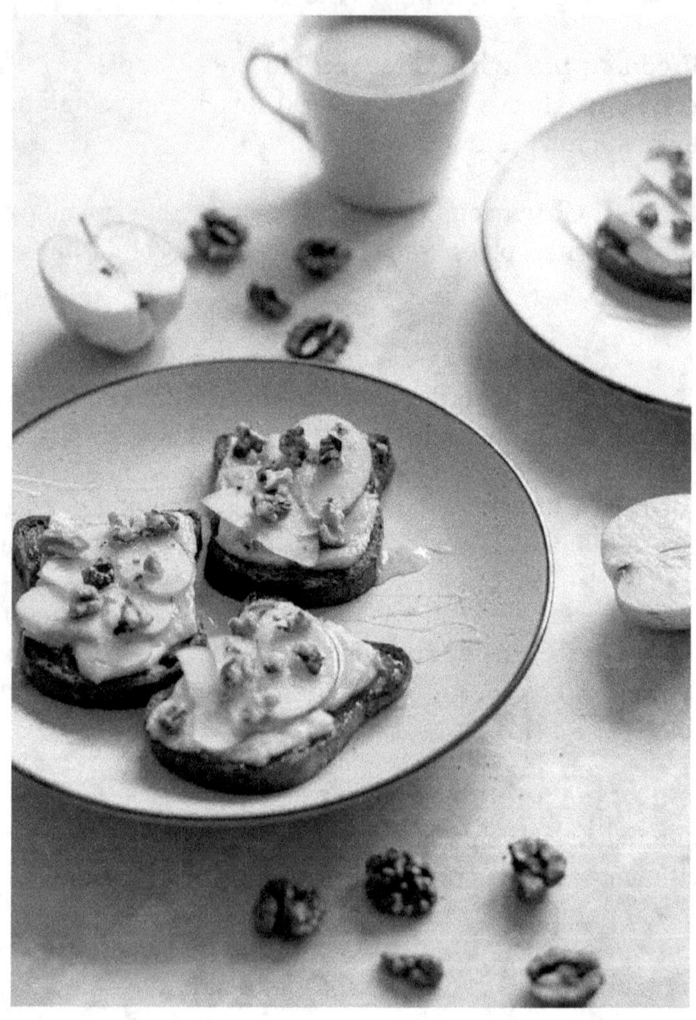

PCOS-Friendly Snacks for Anytime Hunger

Navigating snack choices with PCOS involves finding the right balance of nutrients to keep you energized and satisfied throughout the day. In this chapter, we'll explore practical tips and delicious PCOS-friendly snacks to curb those anytime hunger pangs. The focus is on simplicity, flavor, and nourishment, ensuring you have a variety of snacks at your fingertips that align with your PCOS dietary goals. Let's dive into the world of satisfying and PCOS-friendly snacks.

1. Greek Yogurt Parfait:

Ingredients:

- Greek yogurt (unsweetened)
- Fresh berries (blueberries, strawberries)
- Almonds or walnuts (chopped)
- Drizzle of honey (optional)

Instructions:

A. Arrange fresh berries and Greek yoghurt in a bowl or glass.
B. Sprinkle chopped almonds or walnuts on top.

C. Drizzle with honey for a touch of sweetness if desired.

Why it Works:

I.   Greek yogurt provides protein and probiotics.
II.   Berries offer antioxidants and fiber.
III. Nuts add healthy fats and crunch.

2. Hummus with Veggie Sticks:

Ingredients:

➢ Hummus (store-bought or homemade)
➢ Carrot and cucumber sticks

Instructions:

A. Dip carrot and cucumber sticks into hummus.
B. Enjoy this satisfying and crunchy snack.

Why it Works:

I.   Hummus provides protein and healthy fats.
II.   Carrots and cucumbers offer vitamins and hydration.
III. A balanced combination for a quick and easy snack.

3. Avocado Toast on Whole Grain Crackers:

Ingredients:

- ➤ Whole grain crackers
- ➤ Ripe avocado
- ➤ Cherry tomatoes (sliced)
- ➤ Sprinkle of chia seeds

Instructions:

A. Spread mashed avocado on whole grain crackers.
B. Top with sliced cherry tomatoes and a sprinkle of chia seeds.

Why it Works:

I. Avocado provides healthy fats and fiber.
II. Whole grain crackers offer complex carbohydrates.
III. Tomatoes add flavor and additional nutrients.

4. Cottage Cheese with Pineapple:

Ingredients:

- ➤ Cottage cheese
- ➤ Fresh pineapple (cubed)

Instructions:

    A. Combine cottage cheese with fresh pineapple cubes.

    B. Enjoy this refreshing and protein-packed snack.

Why it Works:

    I.   Cottage cheese is a good source of protein.

    II.   Pineapple adds natural sweetness and vitamin C.

    III.   A simple yet satisfying combination.

5. Trail Mix with Dark Chocolate:

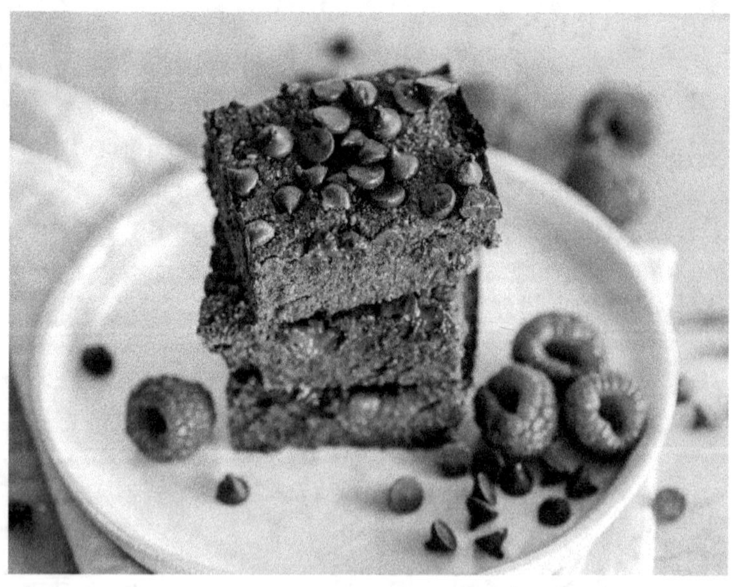

Ingredients:

> ➤ Mixed nuts (almonds, walnuts, cashews)
> ➤ Dried berries (cranberries, blueberries)
> ➤ Dark chocolate chips or chunks

Instructions:

A. Mix nuts, dried berries, and dark chocolate in a bowl.
B. Portion out for a convenient and tasty snack.

Why it Works:

I. Nuts provide healthy fats and protein.
II. Dried berries offer natural sweetness and fibcr.
III. Dark chocolate adds antioxidants and indulgence.

6. Rice Cake with Almond Butter and Banana:

Ingredients:

> ➤ Rice cake (whole grain)
> ➤ Almond butter (unsweetened)
> ➤ Sliced banana

Instructions:

A. Spread almond butter on a rice cake.
B. Top with sliced banana for a satisfying combo.

Why it Works:

I.   The base of rice cakes is crisp and light.
II. Almond butter provides healthy fats and protein.
III. Banana adds natural sweetness and potassium.

7. Veggie Omelette Muffins:

Ingredients:

➢ Eggs
➢ Chopped vegetables (bell peppers, spinach, tomatoes)
➢ Feta or goat cheese (optional)

Instructions:

A. Whisk eggs and mix in chopped vegetables. Fill muffin pans with mixture, and bake until mixture is set.
B. Optional: Add crumbled feta or goat cheese for extra flavor.

Why it Works:

    I.   Eggs are a great source of protein.

   II.   Vegetables offer vitamins and minerals.

 III.   A portable and savory snack option.

8. Quinoa Salad Cups:

Ingredients:

- ➤ Cooked quinoa
- ➤ Diced cucumber, cherry tomatoes, and bell peppers
- ➤ Feta cheese (crumbled)
- ➤ Olive oil and lemon dressing

Instructions:

A. Mix cooked quinoa with diced vegetables and feta cheese.

B. Drizzle with olive oil and lemon dressing.

C. Serve in small cups for a refreshing snack.

Why it Works:

    I.   Quinoa provides protein and complex carbohydrates.

   II.   Vegetables add color, flavor, and nutrients.

 III.   A light and satisfying option for anytime hunger.

9. Chia Seed Pudding:

Ingredients:

- ➤ Chia seeds
- ➤ Almond milk (unsweetened)
- ➤ Vanilla extract
- ➤ Fresh berries for topping

Instructions:

A. Mix chia seeds with almond milk and vanilla extract. To make it thicken, put it in the fridge.
B. Top with fresh berries before serving.

Why it Works:

I. Chia seeds offer fiber and omega-3 fatty acids.
II. Almond milk provides a dairy-free base.
III. A versatile and customizable pudding.

10. Apple Slices with Nut Butter:

Ingredients:

- ➤ Apple (sliced)
- ➤ Nut butter of choice (almond, peanut, or cashew)

Instructions:

    A. Spread nut butter on apple slices.

    B. Enjoy the crispness of apples with the creamy nut butter.

Why it Works:

    I.   Apples offer natural sweetness and fiber.

    II.   Nut butter provides healthy fats and protein.

    III.   A classic and satisfying combination.

Practical Tips for PCOS-Friendly Snacking:

1. Balanced Combinations:

Aim for snacks that combine protein, healthy fats, and carbohydrates to keep you full and satisfied.

2. Portion Control:

Practice mindful portion control to avoid overeating, especially with calorie-dense snacks.

3. Hydration:

Stay hydrated by incorporating water-rich snacks like fresh fruits and vegetables.

4. Prep in Advance:

Prepare snacks in advance to have convenient options readily available, reducing the temptation of less healthy choices.

5. Variety is Key:

Explore a variety of PCOS-friendly snacks to keep your taste buds excited and ensure you receive a range of nutrients.

6. Listen to Your Body:

 Pay attention to the cues your body gives you when it feels hungry or satisfied. Snack when hungry and choose nutrient-dense options.

7. Avoid Highly Processed Snacks:

Limit highly processed snacks that may contain added sugars and unhealthy fats. Instead, choose complete, minimally processed foods.

8. Customize to Your Preferences:

Tailor PCOS-friendly snacks to your preferences and dietary requirements. Experiment with ingredients and flavors that you enjoy.

9. Plan Snacks Around Activities:

Plan snacks around your daily activities to ensure you have energy when needed. For example, have a snack before or after a workout.

10. Keep it Simple:

Snacking doesn't have to be complicated. Keep it simple with easy-to-prep options that fit your nutritional needs.

Conclusion - Snacking Smart with PCOS

Finding the right approach to snacking with PCOS is a journey of balance and understanding. In this chapter, we explored the significance of smart snacking for managing PCOS symptoms and supporting overall health. As you embark on incorporating these insights into your lifestyle, let's summarize the key takeaways and offer some parting thoughts.

Key Takeaways:

Balance is Key: Striking a balance in your snacks helps regulate blood sugar levels, manage weight, and support hormonal balance—essential aspects for individuals with PCOS.

Choose Nutrient-Dense Options: Opt for snacks that are rich in nutrients like fiber, healthy fats, and protein. These choices promote satiety and contribute to overall well-being.

Mindful Portioning: Be mindful of portion sizes to avoid overeating. Portion control is crucial for maintaining a healthy weight and managing insulin resistance associated with PCOS.

Combat Cravings with Healthy Alternatives: Combatting cravings with smart, PCOS-friendly alternatives empowers you to satisfy your snack desires without compromising your health goals.

Hydration Matters: Stay well-hydrated. Often, our bodies can mistake thirst for hunger, so keeping hydrated can help manage unnecessary snacking.

Parting Thoughts:

Navigating snacking with PCOS is about making informed choices that align with your health objectives. Embrace variety in your snacks, experiment with new recipes, and most importantly, listen to your body. PCOS is a unique journey for each individual, and what works well for one person might differ for another. The key is to find a snacking approach that suits your preferences, supports your health, and contributes to your overall well-being.

As you embark on this journey, remember that small changes can lead to significant improvements over time. Celebrate your successes, learn from your experiences, and remain patient with yourself. Snacking smart is not about perfection but about making conscious, sustainable choices that contribute to your health and happiness.

Empower Yourself: A Call to Action

Now armed with knowledge on snacking smart with PCOS, it's time to put this wisdom into action. Create a plan for incorporating nutrient-dense snacks into your daily routine. Experiment with recipes, discover what resonates with your taste buds, and most importantly, enjoy the process of nurturing your body with thoughtful, PCOS-friendly snacks.

Remember, you are on a journey to better health, and every positive choice you make contributes to that journey. Snack smart, savor the flavors, and embrace the empowering path of nourishing yourself with choices that align with your well-being. Here's to your health and vitality!

Guilt-Free Sweet Treats

Satisfying your sweet tooth while staying mindful of PCOS dietary goals is not only possible but also delightful. In this chapter, we'll explore guilt-free sweet treats that bring joy without compromising your commitment to a PCOS-friendly lifestyle. The key is to embrace smart ingredient choices, balance, and portion control. Let's dive into the world of guilt-free indulgence.

1. Dark Chocolate-Covered Strawberries:

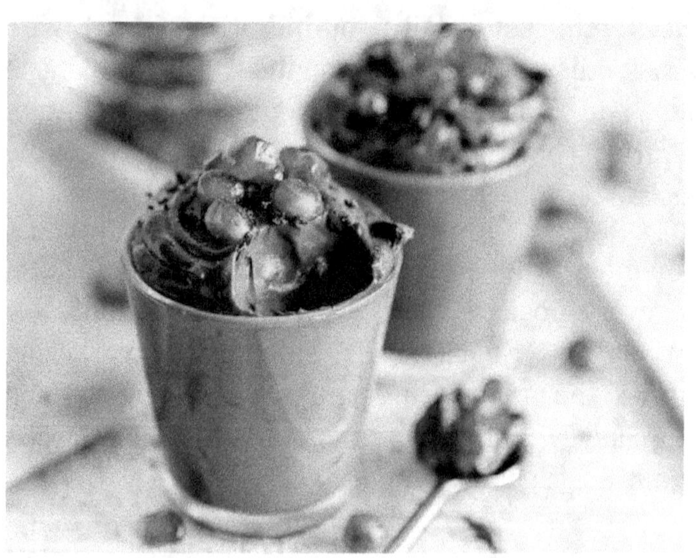

Ingredients:

> ➤ Fresh strawberries
> ➤ Dark chocolate (70% cocoa or higher)

Instructions:

A. Melt dark chocolate in a bowl.
B. Make sure to dip each strawberry into the melted chocolate.
C. Place on parchment paper to set.

Why it Works:

I. Dark chocolate offers antioxidants and indulgence.
II. Strawberries provide natural sweetness and vitamin C.
III. A simple yet decadent treat.

2. Frozen Banana Bites:

Ingredients:

> ➤ Bananas, sliced
> ➤ Almond butter or peanut butter
> ➤ Dark chocolate (melted)

Instructions:

A. Spread almond butter on banana slices.
B. Create banana sandwiches and dip in melted dark chocolate.
C. Freeze until the chocolate sets.

Why it Works:

I. Bananas offer natural sweetness and potassium.
II. Almond butter provides healthy fats and protein.
III. A satisfying frozen treat.

3. Baked Cinnamon Apple Chips:

Ingredients:

➤ Apples, thinly sliced
➤ Cinnamon
➤ Stevia or honey (optional)

Instructions:

A. Preheat the oven and arrange apple slices on a baking sheet.
B. Sprinkle with cinnamon and sweeten with stevia or honey if desired.
C. Bake until crisp.

Why it Works:

I. Apples offer natural sweetness and fiber.
II. Cinnamon adds flavor without added sugar.
III. A crispy, guilt-free substitute for chips.

4. Chia Seed Pudding Parfait:

Ingredients:

➤ Almond milk-based, chia seed pudding
➤ Mixed berries
➤ Granola (unsweetened)

Instructions:

A. Layer chia seed pudding, mixed berries, and granola.
B. Repeat for a visually appealing parfait.

Why it Works:

I. Chia seeds offer omega-3 fatty acids and fiber.
II. Berries provide antioxidants and natural sweetness.
III. Granola adds crunch without excessive sugar.

5. Greek Yogurt Bark:

Ingredients:

➤ Greek yogurt (unsweetened)

> Mixed nuts (almonds, walnuts)
> Dark chocolate chips

Instructions:

A. Mix Greek yogurt with chopped nuts.
B. Transfer the mixture onto a tray coated with parchment.
C. Sprinkle dark chocolate chips on top.
D. Freeze until solid and break into pieces.

Why it Works:

I. Greek yogurt offers protein and probiotics.
II. Nuts provide healthy fats and crunch.
III. Dark chocolate chips add sweetness in moderation.

6. Coconut and Almond Energy Bites:

Ingredients:

> Shredded coconut (unsweetened)
> Almond flour
> Coconut oil (melted)
> Almond extract
> Stevia or honey (optional)

Instructions:

A. Mix shredded coconut, almond flour, melted coconut oil, and almond extract.

B. Add stevia or honey for sweetness if preferred.

C. Roll into bite-sized balls and refrigerate.

Why it Works:

I. Coconut offers healthy fats and sweetness.

II. Almond flour provides protein and texture.

III. A convenient and satisfying energy boost.

7. Avocado Chocolate Mousse:

Ingredients:

- ➤ Ripe avocado
- ➤ Cocoa powder (unsweetened)
- ➤ Vanilla extract
- ➤ Almond milk (unsweetened)
- ➤ Stevia or honey (optional)

Instructions:

A. Blend avocado, cocoa powder, vanilla extract, and almond milk.

B. If desired, add honey or stevia for sweetness.

C. Chill before serving.

Why it Works:

I. Avocado adds creaminess and healthy fats.

II. Without any extra sugar, chocolate flavour is produced by cocoa powder.

III. A luscious and guilt-free chocolate treat.

8. Berry and Yogurt Popsicles:

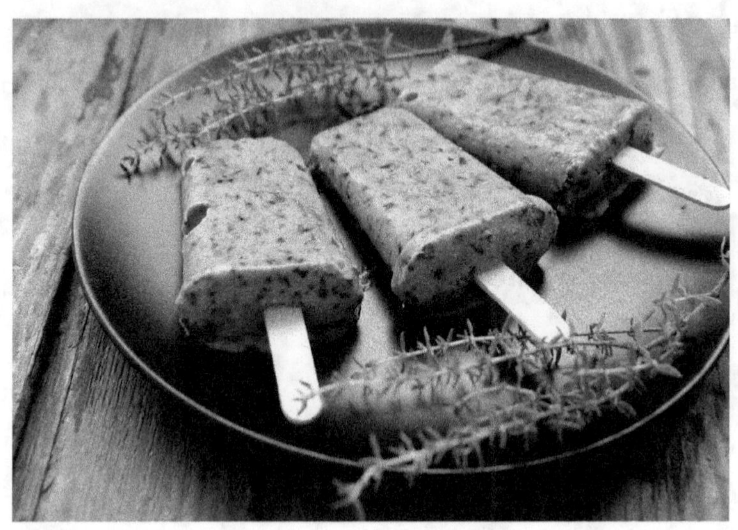

Ingredients:

- ➢ Mixed berries (blueberries, raspberries, strawberries)
- ➢ Greek yogurt (unsweetened)
- ➢ Stevia or honey (optional)

Instructions:

A. Blend berries with a touch of sweetener if desired.
B. Layer berry puree and Greek yogurt in popsicle molds.
C. Freeze until solid.

Why it Works:

    I.   Berries offer antioxidants and natural sweetness.

    II.   Greek yogurt provides protein and creaminess.

    III.   A refreshing and guilt-free frozen treat.

9. Oatmeal Raisin Energy Balls:

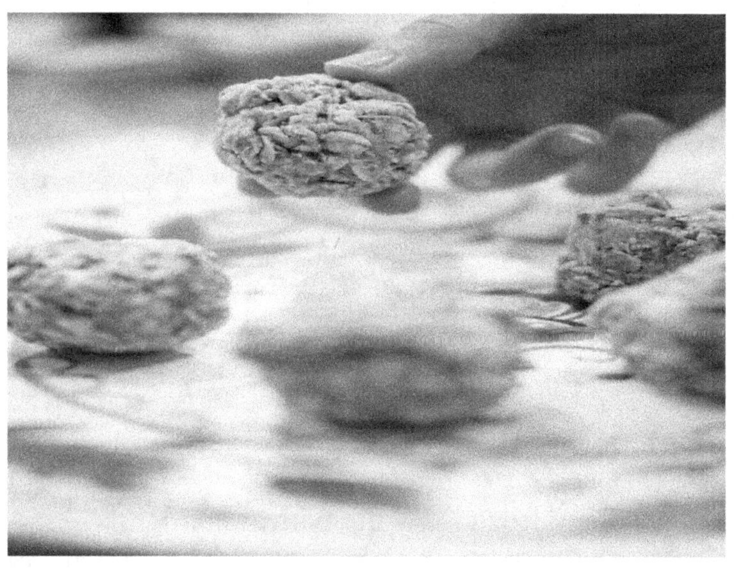

Ingredients:

> Oats (rolled or quick)
> Raisins
> Almond butter
> Vanilla extract
> Cinnamon

Instructions:

A. Mix oats, raisins, almond butter, vanilla extract, and cinnamon.
B. Refrigerate after rolling into bite-sized energy balls.

Why it Works:

I.   Oats offer fiber and sustained energy.
II.   Raisins add natural sweetness.
III. A convenient and satisfying snack.

10. Peach and Almond Sorbet:

Ingredients:

➢ Frozen peaches
➢ Almond milk (unsweetened)
➢ Stevia or honey (optional)

Instructions:

A. Blend frozen peaches with almond milk.
B. You might also use honey or stevia for sweetness.
C. Freeze for a sorbet-like consistency.

Why it Works:

I.   Peaches offer natural sweetness and vitamins.
II.   Almond milk adds creaminess without dairy.

III.   A cool and guilt-free dessert option.

Practical Tips for Enjoying Guilt-Free Sweet Treats:

1. Mindful Portions:

Savor sweet treats in mindful portions to avoid overindulgence.

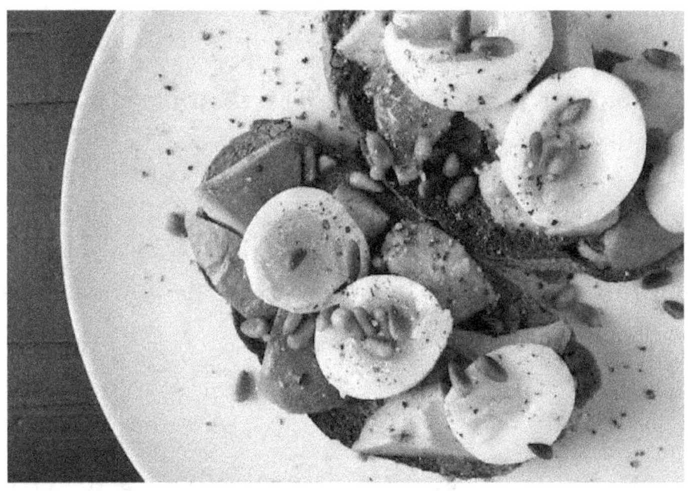

2. Opt for Natural Sweeteners:

Choose natural sweeteners like stevia, honey, or maple syrup instead of refined sugars.

3. Include Protein:

Incorporate protein sources like Greek yogurt, nuts, or nut butter to enhance satiety.

4. Balanced Ingredients:

Aim for a balance of healthy fats, carbohydrates, and protein in your sweet treats for sustained energy.

5. Experiment with Flavors:

Experiment with different flavors and textures to keep your sweet treats exciting and satisfying.

6. Hydration:

Stay hydrated by drinking water alongside sweet treats to support digestion.

7. Customize to Preferences:

Customize recipes based on your taste preferences and dietary requirements.

8. Prepare in Advance:

Prepare guilt-free sweet treats in advance to have convenient and healthier options readily available.

9. Quality Over Quantity:

Choose high-quality ingredients over processed alternatives for a more satisfying and nourishing experience.

10. Share and Enjoy:

Share guilt-free sweet treats with friends or family to enjoy the experience together.

Conclusion: Savoring Sweet Moments without Guilt

Indulging in sweet treats doesn't mean compromising your commitment to a PCOS-friendly lifestyle. These guilt-free options allow you to savor the sweet moments without guilt. As we wrap up our discussion on guilt-free sweet treats, let's reflect on the essence of this journey and offer some final thoughts.

Key Takeaways:

Smart Sweet Swaps: Discovering alternative sweeteners and healthier ingredient options empowers you to create guilt-free sweet treats. From natural sweeteners to nutrient-dense alternatives, these swaps can transform your desserts.

Mindful Moderation: The key to guilt-free indulgence is mindful moderation. Understanding portion control and savoring sweet treats in moderation contributes to both satisfaction and overall well-being.

Balancing Nutrients: Integrating nutrient-dense ingredients into your sweet treats adds a layer of balance. These ingredients not only enhance the nutritional profile but also contribute to better blood sugar management and hormonal balance.

Personalized Treats: Tailoring sweet treats to your preferences ensures that you genuinely enjoy every bite. Experiment with flavors, textures, and ingredients to find what resonates best with your taste buds.

Parting Thoughts: Savoring sweet moments without guilt is about embracing a balanced, sustainable approach to dessert. PCOS-friendly sweet treats aren't just about substituting ingredients but about redefining your relationship with sweets. By making informed choices and relishing each bite consciously, you can enjoy desserts as a delightful part of your lifestyle rather than a source of guilt.

As you venture into creating and enjoying guilt-free sweet treats, remember that it's okay to treat yourself. Celebrate the sweetness of life, share these moments with loved ones, and take pleasure in the journey of nourishing your body with treats that align with your well-being.

Empower Yourself: A Call to Action

Now armed with knowledge on guilt-free sweet treats, it's time to put this wisdom into action.

Experiment with recipes, personalize your desserts to match your preferences, and most importantly, savor the joy of guilt-free indulgence.

As you navigate the world of PCOS-friendly sweet treats, consider sharing your creations with others. You might inspire someone else on their journey to savoring sweet moments without guilt. Remember, it's not just about what you eat but about the positive choices you make to support your health and happiness.

Here's to relishing guilt-free sweet treats, celebrating life's sweetness, and empowering yourself on your PCOS journey. Enjoy every bite, guiltlessly and joyfully!

Balancing Cravings with Fertility Goals

Navigating cravings while staying true to your fertility goals might feel like a delicate dance, but it's a dance you can master. In this chapter, we'll explore practical tips for balancing those cravings with your fertility aspirations. By making informed choices and finding satisfying alternatives, you can indulge in cravings without compromising your overall health. Let's dive into this journey of balance.

Understanding Cravings:

Cravings are a natural part of life and often stem from a combination of emotional, psychological, and physiological factors. While it's okay to indulge occasionally, finding a balance that aligns with your fertility goals is crucial. Here are some practical tips to help you navigate and satisfy those cravings:

1. Listen to Your Body:

Understanding the root cause of your cravings starts with listening to your body. Could it be an emotional trigger or are you genuinely hungry? Pay attention to physical hunger cues, like a growling stomach, and address them with nutrient-dense snacks.

2. Identify Nutrient Deficiencies:

Cravings can sometimes be your body's way of signaling nutrient deficiencies. If you find yourself craving specific foods, consider whether there might be a lack of certain nutrients in your diet. Consult with a healthcare professional to explore any potential deficiencies and adjust your diet accordingly.

3. Opt for Smart Alternatives:

When a craving strikes, opt for smart alternatives that align with your fertility goals. For example, if you're craving something sweet, choose a piece of fruit or a small serving of dark chocolate instead of reaching for highly processed sweets.

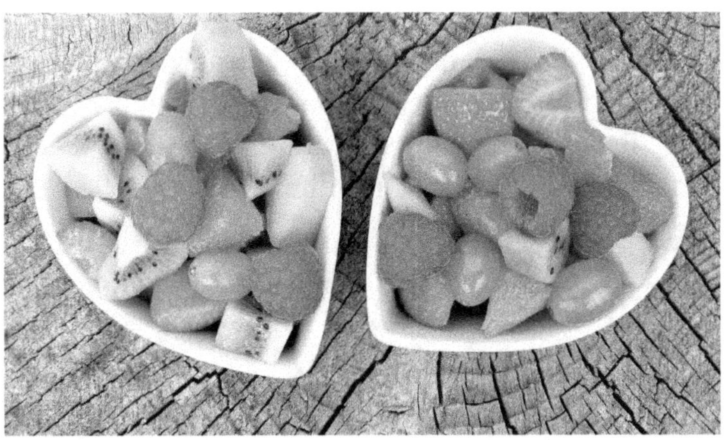

4. Mindful Indulgence:

Allow yourself the pleasure of indulgence in moderation. Instead of completely denying your cravings, enjoy them mindfully and in controlled portions. This approach can help satisfy your desires without derailing your fertility-focused dietary efforts.

5. Stay Hydrated:

Thirst can sometimes be mistaken for hunger, leading to unnecessary cravings.. As the day wears on, make sure you're drinking enough water. When a craving strikes, try drinking a glass of water first and see if it subsides.

6. Plan Balanced Meals:

Strive to plan balanced meals that include a mix of lean proteins, complex carbohydrates, and healthy fats. Balanced meals contribute to overall satiety, reducing the likelihood of intense cravings between meals.

7. Include Variety in Your Diet:

Introduce variety into your diet to minimize the risk of monotony-induced cravings. A diverse range of nutrient-dense foods ensures you obtain a broad spectrum of essential vitamins and minerals.

8. Address Emotional Triggers:

Cravings are not always about physical hunger; they can also be linked to emotions. If stress, boredom, or other emotional triggers contribute to your cravings, find alternative ways to address those emotions. Engaging in activities you enjoy or practicing relaxation techniques can be beneficial.

Balancing Cravings and Fertility Goals:

Balancing cravings with fertility goals involves making conscious choices that prioritize both your short-term desires and long-term aspirations. Here are practical tips for maintaining this equilibrium:

1. Plan Ahead:

Anticipate situations where cravings might arise and plan accordingly. Having fertility-friendly snacks readily available can help you make healthier choices when cravings strike.

2. Educate Yourself:

Understanding the impact of certain foods on fertility can empower you to make informed choices. Educate yourself about fertility-friendly options and incorporate them into your diet.

3. Include Fertility-Boosting Foods:

Integrate fertility-boosting foods into your meals and snacks. Foods rich in antioxidants, omega-3 fatty acids, and key vitamins and minerals support reproductive health and can be part of a satisfying and balanced diet.

4. Seek Professional Guidance:

Consult with a nutritionist or healthcare professional specializing in fertility to create a personalized dietary plan. They can provide insights tailored to your specific needs and goals.

5. Mindful Eating Practices:

Practice mindful eating to enhance your awareness of cravings and the choices you make. Being present during meals helps you savor the flavors and prevents overindulgence.

6. Find Healthier Substitutes:

Identify healthier substitutes for your go-to cravings. Whether it's swapping sugary snacks for fresh fruit or opting for whole grains instead of refined carbs, finding alternatives contributes to a fertility-friendly diet.

7. Keep a Food Journal:

Maintain a food journal to track your cravings, their triggers, and the choices you make. This self-awareness can provide valuable insights into patterns and areas for improvement in your dietary habits.

8. Accountability Partner:

Share your fertility journey with a trusted friend, family member, or partner who can provide support and hold you accountable. Having someone to share your goals and challenges with can make the process more manageable.

Conclusion: Finding Harmony in Cravings and Fertility Goals

Balancing cravings with fertility goals is a dynamic process that requires self-awareness, education, and practical strategies. By understanding your body's signals, making informed choices, and maintaining a fertility-friendly diet, you can find harmony between satisfying your cravings and working towards your long-term reproductive health. Remember, it's not about perfection but about making consistent, mindful choices that support your overall well-being. Embrace the journey, celebrate progress, and continue striving for a balanced and fertility-focused lifestyle.

CHAPTER EIGHT:

BEVERAGES

Stay hydrated and enjoy flavorful beverages that complement your PCOS-friendly lifestyle. Here are practical tips to make mindful choices when it comes to drinks.

Practical Tips:

Infused Water: Enhance your water with slices of citrus fruits, cucumber, or mint for a refreshing and hydrating option without added sugars.

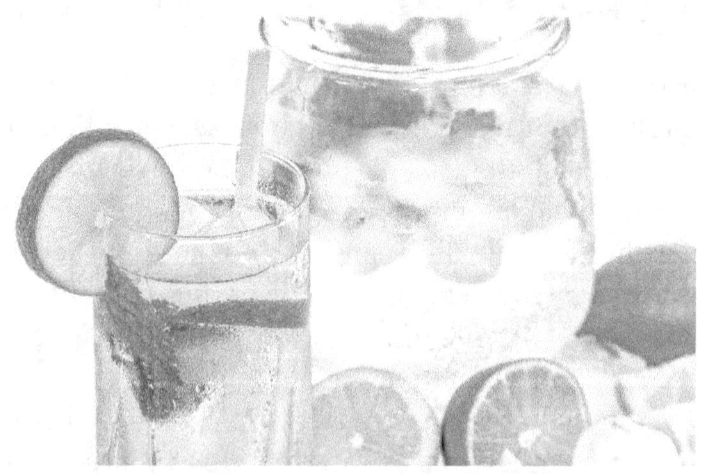

Herbal Teas: Explore a variety of herbal teas like peppermint, chamomile, or ginger. These teas are caffeine-free and can be enjoyed hot or cold.

Green Tea: Rich in antioxidants, green tea can be a great choice. Opt for unsweetened versions to keep it low in added sugars.

Sparkling Water with a Twist: Choose sparkling water and add a splash of natural flavor with a wedge of lemon, lime, or a few berries for a fizzy and satisfying drink.

Smoothies: Blend fruits, greens, and a liquid base like almond milk or water for a nutrient-packed and tasty smoothie.

Freshly Squeezed Juices: Make your fruit juices at home without added sugars. Focus on whole fruits to retain fiber and essential nutrients.

Golden Milk (Turmeric Latte): Combine turmeric with warm milk for a soothing and anti-inflammatory beverage.

Coconut Water: A hydrating option, coconut water is naturally sweet and provides electrolytes.

Vegetable Juice: Mix various vegetables like carrots, celery, and spinach for a nutrient-dense and refreshing drink.

Iced Herbal Tea: Brew herbal tea, let it cool, and serve it over ice for a cool and hydrating alternative.

Be mindful of added sugars in commercial beverages, as excessive sugar intake can impact PCOS symptoms. By incorporating these practical beverage ideas, you can enjoy a variety of flavors while staying hydrated and supporting your overall well-being.

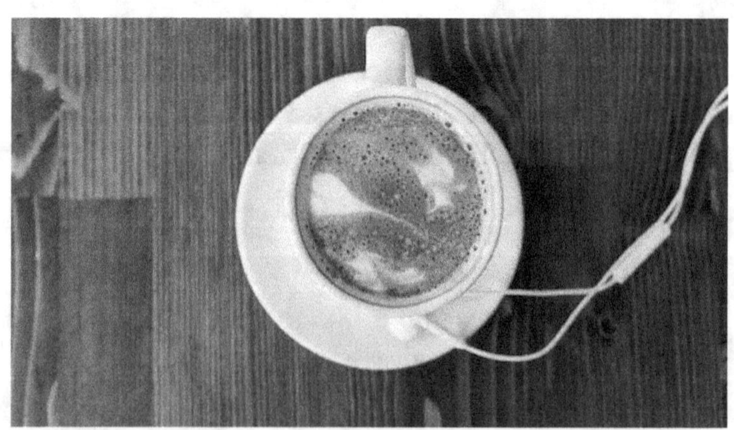

The Importance of Hydration

In the realm of health, few things are as fundamental and often overlooked as the simple act of staying hydrated. In this chapter, we'll dive into the significance of hydration, exploring why it's crucial for overall well-being and particularly beneficial in managing PCOS. Let's keep it straightforward, focusing on clear language and offering practical tips to make hydration a seamless part of your daily routine.

Understanding the Basics:

Why is hydration so vital? At its core, hydration is about maintaining the balance of fluids in our bodies. Water plays a role in nearly every bodily function, from digestion and circulation to temperature regulation and waste elimination. For individuals with PCOS, staying well-hydrated can offer additional benefits.

1. Hormonal Balance:

Adequate hydration supports hormonal balance, a critical aspect for those managing PCOS. Hormones play a key role in the regulation of the menstrual cycle and can be influenced by hydration status. Drinking enough water contributes to hormonal equilibrium, aiding in the management of PCOS symptoms.

2. Blood Sugar Management:

Hydration is closely tied to blood sugar control. For individuals with PCOS, who may experience insulin resistance, maintaining stable blood sugar levels is essential. Water intake can assist in this by supporting insulin sensitivity and helping to manage cravings and overeating.

3. Digestive Health:

Proper hydration is a cornerstone of good digestive health. It facilitates the easy flow of waste through the digestive tract, the breakdown of food, and the absorption of nutrients. For those with PCOS, promoting digestive health is crucial for overall well-being and can contribute to managing symptoms.

Practical Tips for Hydration:

Now that we understand why hydration is vital, let's explore some practical tips to ensure you stay well-hydrated throughout the day:

1. Set a Schedule:

Establish a hydration routine by setting specific times to drink water. Have a glass, for instance, right before bed, right before dinner, and right after you wake up. Creating a schedule helps make hydration a consistent habit.

2. Carry a Reusable Water Bottle:

Carry a reusable water bottle with you all day long. Having water readily available makes it more likely that you'll take regular sips. It's an easy and eco-friendly way to stay hydrated on the go.

3. Infuse with Flavor:

If you're not a fan of plain water, try adding some natural flavours to it. Add slices of citrus fruits, berries, or cucumber to enhance the taste. Herbal teas or diluted fruit juices can also be refreshing alternatives.

4. Monitor Urine Color:

A simple way to gauge your hydration status is by monitoring the color of your urine. Pale yellow to light straw is generally a sign of good hydration, while dark yellow may indicate a need for more fluids.

5. Create Hydration Triggers:

Link hydration to daily activities. For instance, drink a glass of water every time you check your email or each time you take a break. Associating hydration with routine activities helps form a habit.

6. Choose Water-Rich Foods:

Incorporate water-rich foods into your diet. Fruits and vegetables, such as watermelon, cucumber, and oranges, contribute to your overall fluid intake while providing additional nutrients.

7. Listen to Your Body:

Pay attention to your body's signals. Thirst is a clear indication that it's time to drink water. Rather than ignoring this signal, respond to it promptly.

8. Experiment with Temperature:

Some people find it easier to consume water at different temperatures. If you struggle with cold water, try it at room temperature or slightly warm. Herbal teas or infused water can also be enjoyable alternatives.

9. Use Hydration Apps:

Leverage technology by using hydration apps that remind you to drink water throughout the day. These apps can be personalized to your preferences and lifestyle.

10. Gradual Increase:

If you're not accustomed to drinking a lot of water, aim for a gradual increase. Start by adding an extra glass each day until you reach your hydration goals. This prevents overwhelming your system and allows you to adjust comfortably.

Conclusion: Quenching Your Wellness Thirst

Hydration is not just a health task; it's a wellness strategy that can significantly impact your life, especially if you're managing PCOS. By understanding the importance of staying well-hydrated and implementing practical tips, you can turn hydration into a simple, daily habit.

As you embark on this hydration journey, remember that small, consistent efforts lead to lasting changes. Whether it's setting a water-drinking schedule, infusing your water with flavor, or monitoring your urine color, find what works best for you. Cheers to quenching your wellness thirst and embracing the transformative power of staying hydrated!

Fertility-Boosting Beverages

In the quest for optimal fertility, what you drink can be as important as what you eat. This chapter is all about fertility-boosting beverages—simple, everyday drinks that can play a role in supporting reproductive health. Let's keep it straightforward and practical, avoiding complex jargon, as we explore the beverages that can contribute to your fertility journey.

Understanding Fertility-Boosting Beverages:

Before diving into specific drinks, let's understand why certain beverages are considered fertility-boosting:

Hydration and Hormonal Balance:

Adequate hydration is foundational for hormonal balance. Fertility is closely linked to the delicate dance of hormones, and staying well-hydrated supports this intricate system.

Nutrient Intake:

Fertility-boosting beverages often come packed with essential nutrients. These nutrients, ranging from antioxidants to vitamins and minerals, play crucial roles in reproductive health.

Blood Sugar Management:

Stable blood sugar levels are vital for fertility. Some beverages can assist in managing blood sugar, reducing the risk of insulin resistance, which is particularly relevant for those navigating fertility challenges.

Fertility-Boosting Beverage Options:

Now, let's explore practical tips and options for incorporating fertility-boosting beverages into your routine:

1. Water: The Foundation of Fertility: Let's start with the basics—water. Proper hydration supports hormonal balance and aids in overall well-being. Make it a habit to drink ample water throughout the day, and consider infusing it with slices of citrus fruits or cucumber for added flavor.

2. Green Tea: Antioxidant Powerhouse: Antioxidants found in green tea, especially catechins, have been linked to increased fertility. Aim for a moderate intake, as excessive caffeine consumption may have adverse effects.

3. Herbal Infusions: Nettle and Red Clover: Herbal infusions like nettle and red clover are known for their nourishing properties. These caffeine-free options can be a delightful addition to your daily routine. For particular guidance, speak with a medical practitioner.

4. Pomegranate Juice: Rich in Antioxidants: Pomegranate juice is packed with antioxidants, including punicalagins and anthocyanins, which may positively impact fertility. Choose 100% pure pomegranate juice without added sugars for maximum benefits.

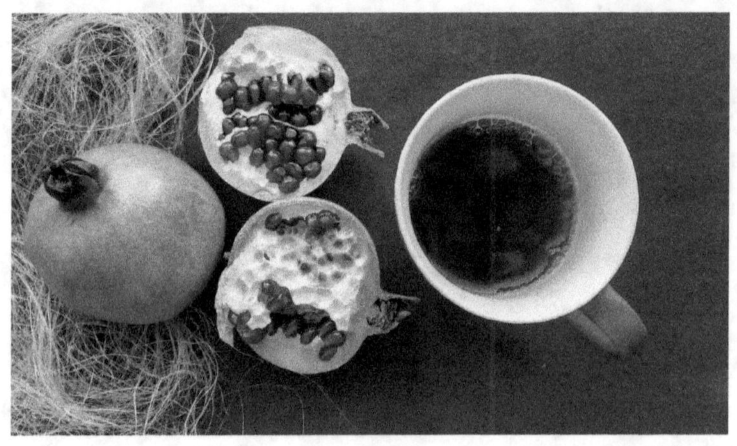

5. Fertility Smoothies: Nutrient-Rich Blends: Create fertility-boosting smoothies by combining nutrient-dense ingredients. Include fruits, leafy greens, Greek yogurt, and fertility-friendly supplements like omega-3 fatty acids or fertility-boosting vitamins.

6. Maca Root Tea: Hormonal Support: For supporting hormonal balance, maca root has long been used. Consider maca root tea as a caffeine-free alternative that may positively influence reproductive health. See a doctor, particularly if you have any pre-existing medical conditions.

7. **Warm Water with Lemon: Alkalizing Elixir:** Starting your day with warm water and lemon can be a gentle alkalizing practice. This simple beverage provides hydration and a dose of vitamin C, supporting both general health and fertility.

8. Coconut Water: Natural Hydration: Coconut water is not only a refreshing beverage but also a natural hydrator rich in electrolytes. It can be a beneficial addition to your fertility-boosting drink choices.

Practical Tips for Incorporating Fertility-Boosting Beverages:

Diversify Your Choices:

Incorporate a variety of fertility-boosting beverages into your routine. This ensures you benefit from a spectrum of nutrients and compounds that support reproductive health.

Limit Caffeine Intake:

While some beverages like green tea offer fertility benefits, excessive caffeine can have adverse effects. Be mindful of your overall caffeine intake and choose decaffeinated options when necessary.

Stay Hydrated Throughout the Day:

Make a conscious effort to stay well-hydrated. Set reminders if needed and carry a reusable water bottle to encourage regular sips.

Consult with a Healthcare Professional:

Before making significant changes to your beverage choices, especially if considering herbal infusions or supplements, consult with a healthcare professional. Personalised recommendations depending on your health situation can be given by them.

Incorporate into Daily Routines:

Make fertility-boosting beverages a seamless part of your daily routine. Whether it's starting your morning with warm lemon water or enjoying a fertility smoothie as an afternoon snack, find ways to integrate these drinks effortlessly.

Conclusion: Sip Your Way to Fertility Wellness:

Fertility-boosting beverages offer a simple yet impactful way to support your reproductive health. By staying well-hydrated and incorporating nutrient-rich drinks into your routine, you can sip your way to fertility wellness. Remember, consistency is key, and small, mindful choices can contribute to your overall fertility journey. Here's to nurturing your body with beverages that align with your fertility goals!

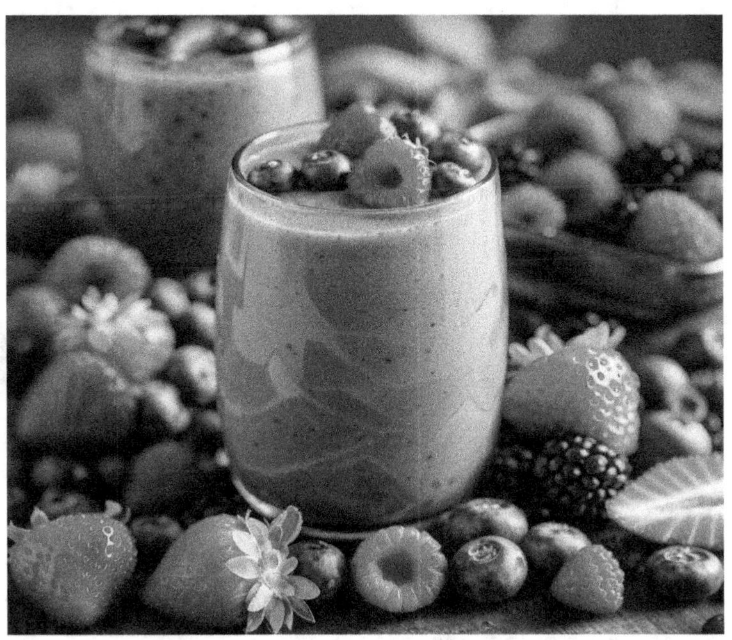

Infused Waters, Teas, and More

Embarking on a journey to enhance your well-being doesn't always require complex solutions. This chapter explores the simple yet powerful world of infused waters, teas, and more—everyday beverages that can elevate your hydration experience. Let's keep it clear, straightforward, and practical as we delve into the art of infusing flavor into your drinks for both pleasure and health.

Infused Waters: A Splash of Refreshment

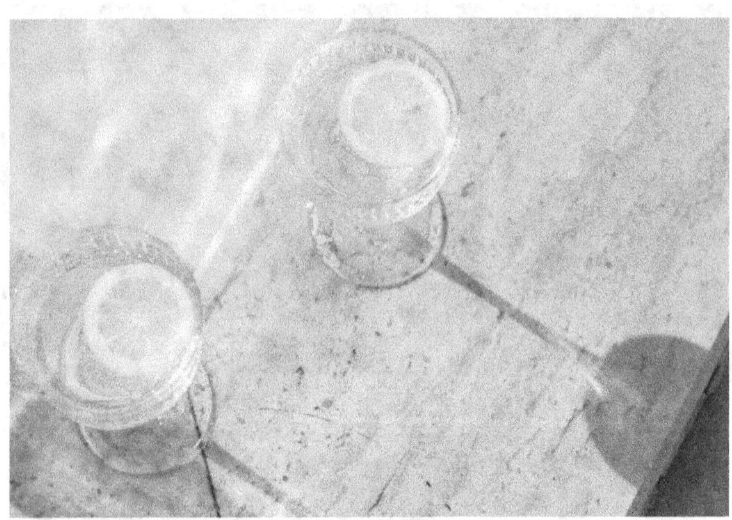

Infused waters are a delightful way to add flavor to your hydration routine. Here are practical tips to create your own refreshing blends:

Simple Combinations:

Start with straightforward combinations like cucumber and mint, lemon and lime, or berries and basil. These pairings not only infuse water with flavor but also bring a burst of natural goodness.

Preparation:

Slice fruits, vegetables, or herbs into manageable pieces to release their flavors. For a stronger infusion, lightly crush herbs like mint or basil to intensify the taste.

Chilled Infusion:

Allow your ingredients to infuse in cold water in the refrigerator for a few hours or overnight. The result is a crisp and flavorful beverage that's perfect for staying cool and hydrated.

Experiment with Seasonal Ingredients:

Embrace seasonal produce to vary your infused water recipes. From citrus fruits in summer to apple and cinnamon in fall, align your choices with what's readily available.

Hydrating with a Twist:

If you enjoy a bit of fizziness, try sparkling water as the base for your infused drinks. The effervescence adds a playful element to your hydration routine.

Teas: A Warm Embrace of Wellness

Teas go beyond a comforting drink—they can be a wellness ritual. Here's how to make the most of teas in your daily routine:

Green Tea for Antioxidants:

Green tea is celebrated for its antioxidant content. Brew a cup and enjoy its earthy flavor while benefiting from the powerful antioxidants that may support overall health.

Herbal Infusions for Relaxation:

Opt for caffeine-free herbal infusions like chamomile or peppermint for a calming experience. These teas are perfect for unwinding after a busy day.

Fertility-Friendly Choices:

Explore fertility-friendly teas like red raspberry leaf tea, which is thought to support reproductive health. For individualised guidance, as always, speak with a healthcare provider.

Customize with Spices:

Elevate your tea experience by adding spices like ginger or cinnamon. Not only do they enhance the flavor, but they also bring additional health benefits.

Time Your Tea:

Align your tea choices with your daily rhythm. For instance, enjoy a calming chamomile tea before bedtime or kickstart your morning with an energizing black or green tea.

More Flavorful Hydration: Beyond the Basics

1. Coconut Water Creations:

Coconut water is not just for sipping on its own. Combine it with slices of tropical fruits like pineapple or kiwi for a hydrating, exotic blend.

2. Aloe Vera Elixir:

Harness the soothing properties of aloe vera by adding it to water. Ensure it's food-grade aloe vera and start with small amounts, gradually adjusting to your taste.

3. Turmeric and Ginger Tonic:

Create a vibrant tonic by infusing water with turmeric slices and ginger. Both ingredients are known for their anti-inflammatory properties.

4. Citrus Zest Infusions:

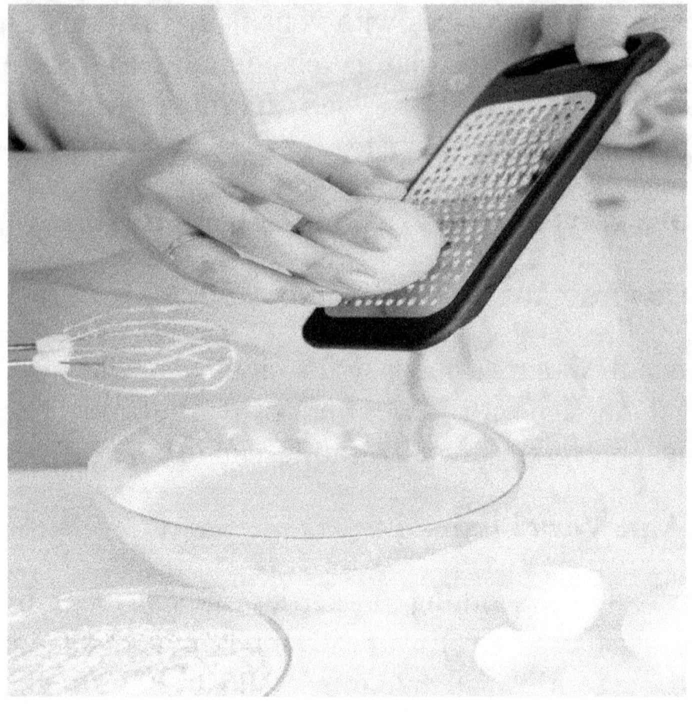

Don't discard citrus peels! Infuse water with citrus zest for a burst of flavor without the acidity of the fruit. It's a clever way to minimize waste and maximize taste.

Practical Tips for Incorporating Flavorful Hydration:

1. Rotate Your Infusions:

Keep things exciting by rotating your infused water and tea choices regularly. This prevents monotony and encourages you to explore a variety of flavors.

2. Prepare Infusions in Batches:

Set aside time to prepare infused waters and teas in larger batches. Having them readily available in the refrigerator makes it easier to stay consistent with your hydration goals.

3. Combine for Complexity:

Experiment with combining infused waters and teas. For instance, pair a berry-infused water with a hibiscus tea for a refreshing and nuanced beverage.

4. Mindful Hydration:

Use your infused beverages as a moment for mindfulness. Take a break, savor the flavors, and let the act of hydrating become a small ritual in your day.

5. Listen to Your Cravings:

Pay attention to your taste preferences and cravings. If you're drawn to certain flavors, tailor your infused drinks accordingly. This ensures that hydration becomes a pleasure rather than a task.

Conclusion: Sip and Savor the Wellness Within

Infused waters, teas, and other flavorful beverages are a delightful gateway to wellness. By infusing your hydration routine with natural flavors, you not only elevate the taste but also add a layer of well-being to each sip. As you explore these simple yet impactful beverages, remember that staying hydrated is not just about meeting a quota—it's about sipping and savoring the wellness within. Cheers to vibrant hydration and the healthful pleasures it brings to your daily life!

CHAPTER NINE:

MANAGING PCOS SYMPTOMS

Effectively managing PCOS symptoms involves a holistic approach. Here are practical tips to navigate the challenges and foster a balanced and healthy lifestyle.

Practical Tips:

Balanced Diet: Adopt a balanced and nutrient-rich diet. Focus on whole foods, lean proteins, and complex carbs to support overall well-being.

Regular Exercise: Engage in regular physical activity. Incorporate a mix of cardiovascular exercises, strength training, and activities you enjoy to promote fitness and manage weight.

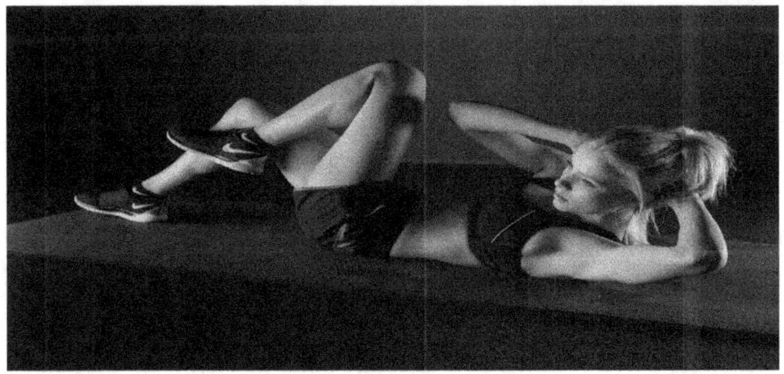

Stress Management: Implement stress-reducing techniques like meditation, deep breathing, or yoga. Managing stress can positively impact hormonal balance.

Adequate Sleep: Prioritize quality sleep. Aim for 7-9 hours per night to support hormonal regulation and overall health.

Regular Check-ups: Schedule regular check-ups with healthcare professionals. Track your hormone levels and take quick action to resolve any issues.

Hydration: Stay well-hydrated. Water is crucial for various bodily functions, including hormone regulation.

Mindful Eating: Practice mindful eating. Pay attention to hunger and fullness cues, and savor each bite for a healthier relationship with food.

Limit Processed Foods: Minimize processed and sugary foods. Opt for whole, unprocessed options to support hormonal balance.

Supplements: Consider supplements under healthcare guidance. Some individuals with PCOS may benefit from supplements like inositol or omega-3 fatty acids.

Support System: Build a strong support system. Share your journey with friends, family, or support groups to receive encouragement and understanding.

Managing PCOS symptoms is a dynamic process. Small, consistent lifestyle changes can contribute to significant improvements over time. By incorporating these practical tips, you empower yourself to navigate the complexities of PCOS and foster a healthier, more balanced life.

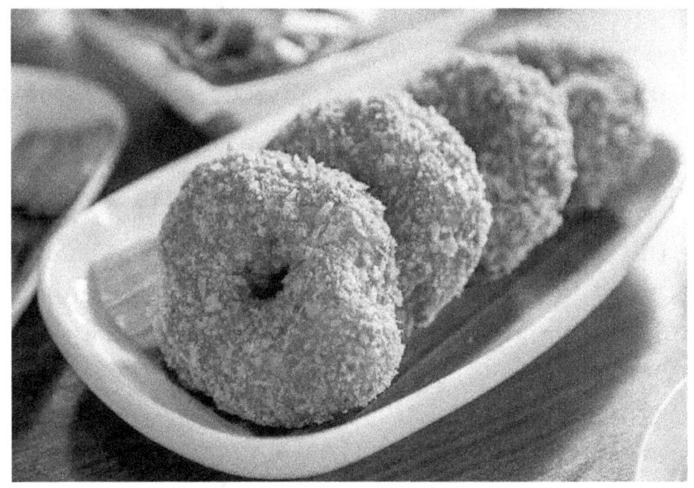

Strategies for Managing PCOS Symptoms Through Diet

Navigating the landscape of Polycystic Ovary Syndrome (PCOS) can be challenging, but your dietary choices play a pivotal role in managing its symptoms. In this chapter, we'll explore straightforward strategies to empower you on your journey to managing PCOS through diet. Let's keep it clear, practical, and easy to understand as we delve into actionable tips that can make a significant difference in your daily life.

Understanding PCOS and Its Dietary Impact:

PCOS is a hormonal disorder that can affect various aspects of health, including menstrual cycles, fertility, and metabolism. While there's no one-size-fits-all solution, adopting a mindful approach to your diet can help alleviate symptoms and promote overall well-being.

1. Embrace Balanced Meals:

Aim for well-balanced meals with a range of fruits and vegetables, whole grains, lean meats, and healthy fats.

Balanced meals contribute to stable blood sugar levels, which is crucial for individuals with PCOS, especially those managing insulin resistance.

2. Prioritize Complex Carbohydrates:

Opt for complex carbohydrates like whole grains, legumes, and sweet potatoes over refined carbohydrates. These choices have a gentler impact on blood sugar levels.

Whole grains like quinoa, brown rice, and oats provide essential nutrients and fiber, supporting digestive health.

3. Incorporate Lean Proteins:

Include lean protein sources such as poultry, fish, tofu, and legumes in your meals. Protein helps with satiety and can assist in managing weight, a common concern for individuals with PCOS.

4. Healthy Fats for Hormonal Balance:

Add avocados, almonds, seeds, and olive oil—among the foods high in healthy fats—to your diet. Healthy fats play a role in hormonal balance, a key consideration for those with PCOS.

5. Mindful Portion Control:

Practice mindful portion control to avoid overeating. Pay attention to hunger and fullness cues, and be conscious of portion sizes to support weight management.

6. Regular, Balanced Snacking:

Incorporate balanced snacks between meals to maintain steady energy levels. Opt for nutrient-dense options like Greek yogurt with berries, a handful of nuts, or carrot sticks with hummus.

7. Hydration for Hormonal Support:

 To stay properly hydrated, make sure you consume enough water throughout the day. Proper hydration supports hormonal balance and aids in overall health, contributing to the management of PCOS symptoms.

8. Choose Whole, Unprocessed Foods:

Prioritize whole, unprocessed foods over highly processed options. Whole foods are rich in nutrients and provide sustained energy, promoting overall health.

9. Limit Added Sugars:

Be mindful of added sugars in your diet. An excessive sugar diet may be a factor in insulin resistance. Examine food labels and select items with the fewest added sugars.

10. Experiment with Anti-Inflammatory Foods:

Incorporate anti-inflammatory foods into your diet, such as fatty fish, berries, turmeric, and leafy greens. These foods may help manage inflammation, a factor in PCOS.

11. Consider Supplements with Professional Guidance:

Consult with a healthcare professional to determine if specific supplements, such as inositol or omega-3 fatty acids, could benefit your PCOS management. Avoid self-prescription and seek personalized advice.

12. Mind-Body Connection:

Acknowledge the mind-body connection in managing PCOS. Incorporate stress-reducing practices like meditation, yoga, or deep breathing exercises into your routine.

13. Regular Physical Activity:

Engage in regular physical activity. Exercise not only supports weight management but also has positive effects on insulin sensitivity and hormonal balance.

14. Individualized Approach:

Recognize that PCOS manifests differently in individuals. A person's solution may not be the solution for another. Listen to your body and tailor your diet to your unique needs.

Conclusion: Your Personalized Approach to PCOS Management

Managing PCOS through diet is not about restriction but about making informed, sustainable choices that support your well-being. By embracing a balanced, mindful approach to eating, you can navigate the complexities of PCOS with greater ease. Remember, it's your journey, and finding what works for you may involve some experimentation. Consult with healthcare professionals, stay attuned to your body, and empower yourself with the knowledge to make choices that contribute to your overall health and happiness. Here's to your journey of managing PCOS through thoughtful, practical dietary strategies!

Weight Management and PCOS

Navigating weight management with Polycystic Ovary Syndrome (PCOS) can pose unique challenges, but practical strategies can make a significant difference. In this chapter, we'll explore straightforward tips to help you manage your weight effectively while living with PCOS. Let's keep it clear, practical, and easy to understand as we delve into actionable steps that align with your health goals.

Understanding the Link Between PCOS and Weight:

PCOS and weight management often go hand in hand, as hormonal imbalances in PCOS can contribute to weight gain and make weight loss more challenging. However, adopting the right strategies can positively impact both PCOS symptoms and overall well-being.

1. Focus on Balanced Nutrition:

Prioritize balanced meals that include a mix of lean proteins, whole grains, healthy fats, and a variety of fruits and vegetables.

Balancing macronutrients helps regulate blood sugar levels, which is crucial for weight management in individuals with PCOS.

2. Choose Whole, Unprocessed Foods:

Opt for whole, unprocessed foods over processed alternatives. Whole foods provide essential nutrients, support satiety, and contribute to overall health.

3. Mindful Portion Control:

Practice mindful portion control to avoid overeating. Listen to your body's hunger and fullness cues, and be conscious of portion sizes to support weight management.

4. Include Lean Proteins:

Incorporate lean protein sources such as poultry, fish, tofu, and legumes in your diet. Protein aids in maintaining muscle mass, which is important for metabolism.

5. Prioritize Complex Carbohydrates:

Sweet potatoes, lentils, and whole grains are good sources of complex carbs. These options provide sustained energy and have a gentler impact on blood sugar levels.

6. Stay Hydrated:

Drink enough water throughout the day to stay well-hydrated. Proper hydration supports metabolism and can contribute to weight management.

7. Limit Added Sugars:

Be mindful of added sugars in your diet. Consuming too much sugar might increase the risk of weight gain and insulin resistance. Check food labels and opt for minimally processed options.

8. Regular Physical Activity:

Engage in regular physical activity. Exercise is a key component of weight management for individuals with PCOS, promoting calorie expenditure and enhancing insulin sensitivity.

9. Set Realistic Goals:

Set achievable and realistic weight management goals. Contrary to harsh, temporary solutions, small, lasting adjustments have a higher chance of being successful in the long run.

10. Consider Professional Guidance:

Consult with healthcare professionals, including a registered dietitian or nutritionist, to develop a personalized nutrition plan. Professional guidance can provide tailored strategies based on your unique needs.

11. Embrace a Variety of Exercises:

Incorporate a mix of aerobic and strength-training exercises. Both types of exercise contribute to overall fitness and can aid in weight management.

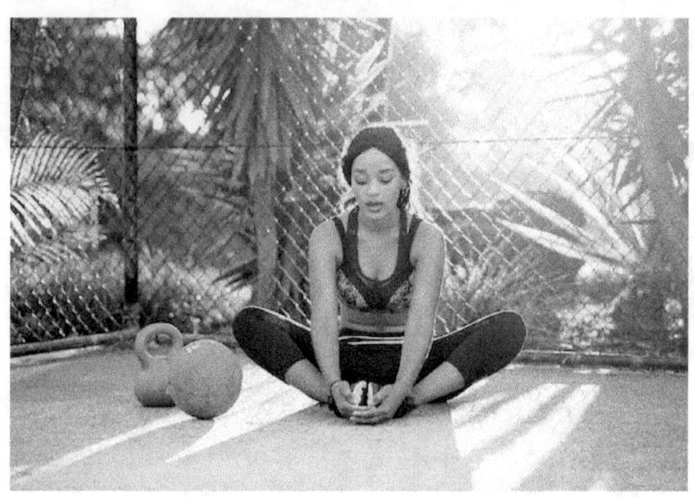

12. Mind-Body Connection:

Acknowledge the mind-body connection in weight management. Stress can impact weight and exacerbate PCOS symptoms, so incorporating stress-reducing practices like meditation or yoga can be beneficial.

13. Monitor Progress Without Obsession:

Keep track of your progress, but avoid obsessive monitoring. Sustainable weight management is a gradual process, and focusing on overall health is more important than a number on the scale.

14. Supportive Lifestyle Changes:

Consider adopting lifestyle changes that support weight management, such as improving sleep quality, managing stress, and fostering a positive relationship with food.

15. Seek Social Support:

Make contact with people who might be travelling a similar path. Social support can provide encouragement, motivation, and a sense of community as you navigate weight management with PCOS.

Conclusion: A Holistic Approach to Weight Management

Managing weight with PCOS is about adopting a holistic approach that considers nutrition, physical activity, and overall well-being. By making informed, sustainable choices and seeking support from healthcare professionals, you can navigate weight management effectively. Remember, your journey is unique, and finding what works for you involves patience and persistence. Here's to embracing a balanced, practical approach to weight management and achieving your health goals with PCOS!

Recipes and Meal Plans for Specific PCOS Symptoms

Navigating the world of recipes and meal plans can be a powerful tool in managing specific symptoms associated with Polycystic Ovary Syndrome (PCOS). In this chapter, we'll explore straightforward and practical recipes tailored to address common PCOS symptoms. Let's keep it clear, simple, and easy to understand as we dive into meals that align with your health goals.

Understanding PCOS Symptom Management Through Nutrition:

PCOS manifests in various ways, and nutritional choices can play a crucial role in addressing specific symptoms. Whether you're dealing with insulin resistance, hormonal imbalances, or weight management, these recipes and meal plans are designed with your well-being in mind.

1. Recipe: Balanced Breakfast Bowl

Ingredients:

- ➤ 1/2 cup cooked quinoa
- ➤ 1/4 cup Greek yogurt
- ➤ 1/2 cup mixed berries (blueberries, strawberries)

➤ 1 tablespoon chia seeds

➤ Drizzle of honey or maple syrup (optional)

Instructions:

A. Combine cooked quinoa and Greek yogurt in a bowl.

B. Top with mixed berries and sprinkle chia seeds.

C. Drizzle with honey or maple syrup if desired.

D. Enjoy this balanced breakfast that provides protein, fiber, and antioxidants.

2. Meal Plan: Hormone-Balancing Lunch

Lunch Option: Quinoa and Chickpea Salad

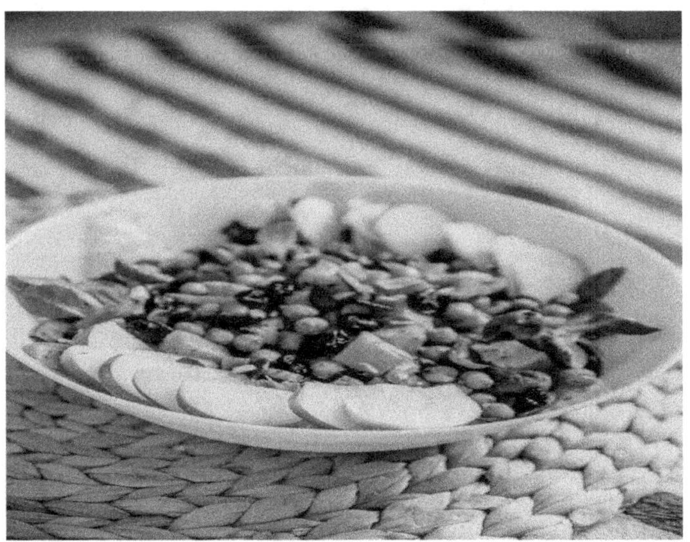

Ingredients:

- ➢ 1 cup cooked quinoa
- ➢ 1/2 cup chickpeas (canned, drained)
- ➢ 1 cup cherry tomatoes, halved
- ➢ 1/4 cup cucumber, diced
- ➢ 2 tablespoons feta cheese
- ➢ Fresh herbs (mint, parsley)
- ➢ Olive oil and lemon dressing

Instructions:

A. Combine cooked quinoa, chickpeas, cherry tomatoes, cucumber, and feta cheese in a bowl.
B. Toss with fresh herbs and drizzle with olive oil and lemon dressing.
C. This lunch is rich in fiber, protein, and healthy fats.

3. Recipe: Insulin-Resistant-Friendly Dinner

Ingredients:

- ➢ Baked salmon fillet
- ➢ Steamed broccoli
- ➢ 1/2 cup quinoa or brown rice
- ➢ Lemon wedges
- ➢ Olive oil for drizzling

Instructions:

A. Bake salmon with a sprinkle of herbs or spices.
B. Steam broccoli until tender-crisp.
C. Serve salmon and broccoli over a bed of quinoa or brown rice.
D. Drizzle with olive oil and squeeze fresh lemon over the dish.
E. This dinner is a balance of omega-3 fatty acids, lean protein, and complex carbohydrates.

4. Meal Plan: Weight Management-Focused Snacks

Snack Options:

➢ Handful of almonds with a small apple
➢ Greek yogurt with a sprinkle of granola
➢ Sliced cucumber with hummus

Instructions:

These snacks are nutrient-dense, providing a mix of protein, healthy fats, and fiber to support satiety.

5. Recipe: Anti-Inflammatory Smoothie

Ingredients:

- ➤ 1 cup spinach
- ➤ 1/2 cup pineapple chunks
- ➤ 1/2 banana
- ➤ 1 tablespoon chia seeds
- ➤ 1 cup coconut water

Instructions:

A. Blend spinach, pineapple, banana, chia seeds, and coconut water until smooth.
B. This smoothie is rich in anti-inflammatory ingredients and hydrating coconut water.

6. Meal Plan: Balanced Day for PCOS Symptom Management

Breakfast:

A. Balanced Breakfast Bowl (as mentioned above)
B. Lunch:
C. Quinoa and Chickpea Salad (as mentioned above)
D. Snack:
E. Greek yogurt with a sprinkle of granola

Dinner:

Baked Salmon Fillet with Steamed Broccoli and Quinoa.

Instructions:

This day provides a variety of nutrients to address hormonal imbalances, insulin resistance, and support weight management.

Practical Tips for Implementing PCOS-Focused Recipes and Meal Plans:

Preparation is Key: Make a plan for your meals and snacks in advance to make sure you have everything you need.

Variety is Vital:

Incorporate a variety of fruits, vegetables, lean proteins, and whole grains to ensure a diverse range of nutrients.

Listen to Your Body: Keep an eye on how your body reacts to various foods. If certain ingredients agree with you, incorporate them into your regular meals.

Stay Hydrated: Water is essential for overall health. Stay hydrated throughout the day to support digestion and nutrient absorption.

Consult with Professionals: Before making significant changes to your diet, especially if you have specific dietary restrictions or health conditions, consult with a registered dietitian or healthcare professional.

Conclusion: Nourishing Your Body with Purpose

These recipes and meal plans are crafted with the intention of supporting your well-being as you navigate the complexities of PCOS. By nourishing your body with purpose and incorporating balanced, nutrient-dense meals, you empower yourself to manage specific symptoms effectively. Remember, it's about making sustainable choices that align with your health goals and contribute to your overall wellness. As you embark on this journey of incorporating PCOS-focused recipes and meal plans into your lifestyle, keep in mind the importance of balance, variety, and personalized choices.

Recognize that each person's experience with PCOS is unique, and what works well for one individual may differ for another. Listen to your body, observe how it responds to different foods, and make adjustments based on your personal preferences and needs.

Moreover, remember that managing PCOS is a holistic endeavor that encompasses not only your dietary choices but also lifestyle factors, such as stress management, sleep, and regular physical activity. Strive for a balanced approach that addresses various aspects of your well-being.

In your pursuit of a healthier, more fulfilling life with PCOS, seek support from healthcare professionals, including registered dietitians, who can provide personalized guidance based on your individual circumstances.

Ultimately, this chapter serves as a starting point—a resource to inspire and guide you in creating meals that align with your health goals. Embrace the journey of discovering what works best for you, and celebrate the positive steps you take toward improved well-being.

Here's to nourishing your body with purpose, making informed choices, and finding joy in the process of caring for yourself. May these recipes and meal plans contribute not only to the management of specific PCOS symptoms but also to a greater sense of vitality, balance, and empowerment in your daily life.

CHAPTER 10:

POST-IVF AND BEYOND

Entering the post-IVF phase is a significant transition. Here are practical tips to guide you through this period and beyond, fostering well-being and embracing the future.

Practical Tips:

Self-Care Rituals: Prioritize self-care. Incorporate rituals that bring comfort, joy, and relaxation into your daily routine.

Emotional Support: Seek emotional support from loved ones or professional counselors. Processing the emotional aspects of the post-IVF journey is crucial.

Maintain a Healthy Lifestyle: Continue with the healthy habits developed during IVF. A balanced diet, regular exercise, and sufficient sleep support overall well-being.

Reflection and Adjustment: Reflect on your journey. Understand that outcomes may vary, and it's okay to adjust expectations. Celebrate the progress made.

Connection with Partner: Nurture your connection with your partner. Open communication is essential during this phase to navigate shared emotions and plans for the future.

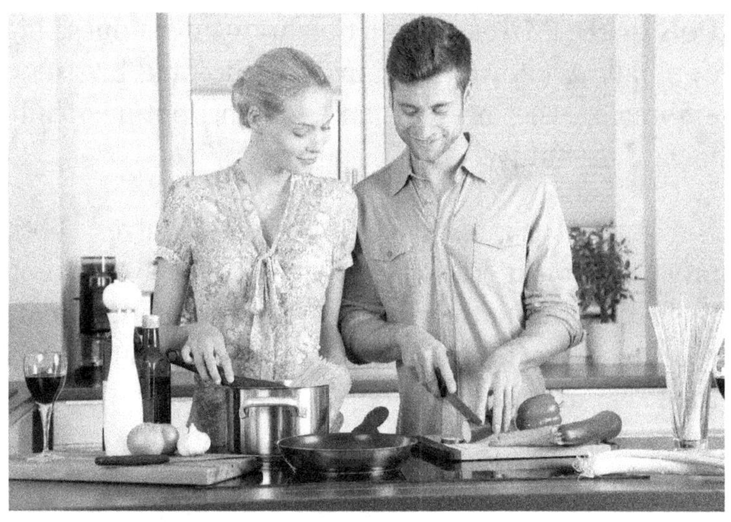

Explore Alternative Paths: Be open to exploring alternative paths to parenthood. Adoption, surrogacy, or other options may be considerations for your family-building journey.

Set New Goals: Establish new goals and aspirations. Whether related to family planning, career, or personal growth, setting new objectives provides direction and purpose.

Regular Check-ups: Maintain regular check-ups with healthcare providers. Monitoring your health remains important for your overall well-being.

Join Support Communities: Connect with others who have gone through similar experiences. Support communities provide understanding and shared insights.

Celebrate Milestones: Celebrate milestones, big or small. Acknowledge your resilience and progress, embracing the present and looking optimistically toward the future.

Navigating the post-IVF period involves both practical considerations and emotional well-being. By incorporating these tips, you lay a foundation for continued growth, resilience, and fulfillment beyond the IVF journey.

Post-IVF Dietary Considerations

Embarking on the post-IVF journey is a significant step in your fertility and wellness path. As you navigate this crucial phase, your dietary choices play a vital role in supporting a healthy pregnancy and recovery. In this chapter, we'll delve into practical and straightforward tips for post-IVF dietary considerations. Let's keep it clear, simple, and focused on empowering you during this important period.

Understanding the Importance of Post-IVF Nutrition:

After undergoing In Vitro Fertilization (IVF), your body has undergone a remarkable process, and providing it with the right nutrients is essential for both recovery and supporting a potential pregnancy. Here are practical considerations to guide your post-IVF dietary choices.

1. Prioritize Nutrient-Rich Foods:

Emphasize a variety of nutrient-dense foods, including fruits, vegetables, whole grains, lean proteins, and healthy fats. These provide the essential vitamins and minerals crucial for overall health.

2. Adequate Protein Intake:

Protein is a cornerstone of post-IVF nutrition. Include sources such as poultry, fish, beans, and dairy products to support tissue repair and development.

3. Essential Fats for Hormonal Health:

Add healthy fat-containing foods such as avocados, nuts, seeds, and olive oil. These fats play a role in hormonal balance, which is particularly crucial during early pregnancy.

4. Hydration is Key:

Stay well-hydrated by drinking plenty of water. Proper hydration supports various bodily functions, aids digestion, and contributes to overall well-being.

5. Mindful Caloric Intake:

While it's essential to nourish your body, be mindful of your caloric intake. Aim for a balanced diet that meets your energy needs without excessive calorie consumption.

6. Consider Folate-Rich Foods:

Folate is crucial for early fetal development. Include foods rich in folate, such as leafy greens, lentils, and fortified cereals, to support the potential early stages of pregnancy.

7. Incorporate Iron-Rich Foods:

Iron is vital for preventing anemia, which can be a concern during pregnancy. Lean meats, beans, and dark, leafy greens are among the foods high in iron that you should eat.

8. Monitor Caffeine Intake:

While moderate caffeine consumption is generally considered safe, it's advisable to monitor your intake. Some studies suggest limiting caffeine during pregnancy, so consider switching to decaffeinated options if needed.

9. Support Digestive Health:

Probiotics from yogurt, kefir, and fermented foods can support digestive health. Pregnancy hormones can affect digestion, and maintaining a healthy gut is beneficial.

10. Diversify Your Plate:

Create well-balanced meals by incorporating a variety of food groups. A diverse diet helps ensure you receive a broad spectrum of nutrients necessary for both your well-being and potential pregnancy.

11. Mind-Body Connection:

Acknowledge the mind-body connection. Practices such as meditation, deep breathing, or gentle exercises can help manage stress and support overall well-being.

12. Plan for Balanced Snacks:

Keep nutrient-rich snacks on hand, such as fresh fruit, nuts, or yogurt. Balanced snacks help maintain steady energy levels throughout the day.

13. Communicate with Your Healthcare Provider:

Talk to your doctor about any dietary restrictions or worries. Personalised advice can be given by them depending on your needs and current state of health.

14. Adequate Prenatal Supplementation:

Continue taking any prenatal supplements recommended by your healthcare provider. These supplements fill nutritional gaps and provide essential nutrients crucial during early pregnancy.

15. Listen to Your Body:

Pay attention to your body's cues and cravings. These can provide insights into your nutritional needs during this unique phase.

Conclusion: Nourishing Your Post-IVF Journey

As you navigate the post-IVF phase, remember that each person's journey is unique. Nourishing your body with purpose and intention can contribute not only to your recovery but also to the potential success of your fertility journey.

This chapter serves as a guide—a roadmap to making informed and practical dietary choices during the post-IVF period. Embrace the opportunity to nourish yourself, support your body, and lay the foundation for a healthy and thriving pregnancy.

May your post-IVF journey be filled with hope, well-being, and the promise of new beginnings. Here's to nourishing your body and nurturing your dreams of building a family.

Maintaining a Healthy Diet for Ongoing Fertility and Overall Well-Being

Congratulations on reaching this stage of your fertility journey. Whether you're actively trying to conceive or simply prioritizing your overall well-being, maintaining a healthy diet is a fundamental aspect of supporting ongoing fertility. In this chapter, we'll explore practical tips and clear guidance to help you nourish your body for sustained fertility and overall health.

Understanding the Role of Diet in Ongoing Fertility:

Your diet plays a crucial role not only in fertility but also in supporting your overall health. As you consider the broader picture of your well-being, here are practical tips to guide you in maintaining a healthy diet.

1. Prioritize a Balanced Plate:

Build meals that include a variety of food groups, focusing on whole grains, lean proteins, healthy fats, and a rainbow of fruits and vegetables. This ensures you receive a broad spectrum of nutrients necessary for fertility and overall health.

2. Lean Proteins for Reproductive Health:

Add in foods high in lean protein, such as fish, poultry, tofu, and lentils. Protein is essential for reproductive health and provides the building blocks for hormones.

3. Incorporate Omega-3 Fatty Acids:

Add foods high in omega-3 fatty acids, like walnuts, flaxseeds, chia seeds, and fatty fish (like mackerel and salmon). These fats support hormonal balance and reproductive health.

4. Fiber-Rich Foods for Digestive Health:

Ensure an ample intake of fiber from whole grains, fruits, vegetables, and legumes. Fiber promotes digestive health, helps regulate hormones, and supports overall well-being.

5. Hydration for Optimal Functioning:

Stay well-hydrated by drinking plenty of water. Proper hydration is essential for overall bodily functions, including reproductive health.

6. Antioxidant-Rich Choices:

Choose foods rich in antioxidants, such as berries, dark leafy greens, and colorful vegetables.

Antioxidants help combat oxidative stress, which can impact fertility.

7. Mindful Caffeine Consumption:

If you consume caffeine, do so in moderation. While it's widely accepted that a modest amount of caffeine is harmless, too much of it can affect fertility.

8. Whole Foods Over Processed Options:

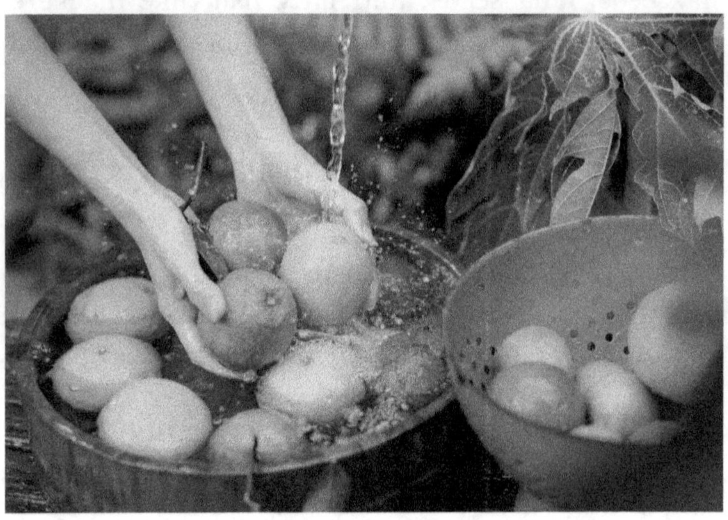

Choose whole, unprocessed foods over those that have undergone extensive processing. Whole foods provide a more comprehensive range of nutrients that support overall health and fertility.

9. Moderate Alcohol Consumption:

If you decide to drink, make sure you do so sparingly. Excessive alcohol intake can affect reproductive hormones, so it's advisable to limit alcohol consumption.

10. Plan Well-Balanced Meals:

Structure your meals to include a balance of macronutrients (carbohydrates, proteins, fats) and micronutrients. This approach supports stable energy levels and provides essential nutrients.

11. Folate and B Vitamins:

Ensure adequate intake of folate and B vitamins. These nutrients play a crucial role in reproductive health and are often recommended for women trying to conceive.

12. Regular Physical Activity:

Engage in regular physical activity. Exercise not only supports overall health but also contributes to hormonal balance and fertility.

13. Consider Prenatal Supplements:

Even if you're not actively trying to conceive, consider continuing with a prenatal supplement. Prenatal vitamins provide additional support for reproductive health and fill potential nutritional gaps.

14. Manage Stress Through Nutrition:

Choose foods that help manage stress, such as those rich in magnesium (leafy greens, nuts, seeds) and vitamin C (citrus fruits, strawberries).

15. Regular Health Check-ups:

Schedule regular health check-ups with your healthcare provider. Monitoring your overall health ensures early detection of any issues that may impact fertility.

Practical Tips for Implementing a Healthy Diet:

Meal Planning: Make a food plan in advance to guarantee a well-rounded and nourishing diet.

Variety is Key:

Incorporate a variety of foods to ensure you receive a broad range of nutrients.

Listen to Your Body:

Make dietary adjustments based on your observations of how your body reacts to various meals.

Stay Informed:

Stay informed about nutritional needs specific to fertility and overall health.

Consult with Professionals:

Consult with a registered dietitian or healthcare provider for personalized advice based on your individual needs.

Conclusion: Nourishing Your Fertility Journey

Maintaining a healthy diet for ongoing fertility and overall well-being is a proactive and empowering step in your journey. By making informed, practical choices, you not only support your reproductive health but also lay the foundation for a vibrant and fulfilling life.

Here's to nourishing your body, embracing your fertility journey with confidence, and fostering a state of well-being that extends far beyond the realms of conception. May your path be filled with vitality, balance, and the joy of nourishing yourself with purpose.

Support and Resources for Your Fertility Journey

Embarking on a fertility journey is a significant undertaking, and having the right support and resources can make a world of difference. In this chapter, we'll explore practical tips and accessible resources to guide you through your fertility journey. Let's keep it straightforward and empower you with the tools you need for support.

Understanding the Importance of Support:

Facing the challenges and uncertainties of a fertility journey can be both emotionally and physically demanding. Having a strong support system and access to valuable resources can provide comfort, guidance, and a sense of community. Here are practical tips to help you navigate this important aspect of your journey.

1. Build a Support Network:

Surround yourself with understanding and supportive individuals. Share your journey with trusted friends and family members who can offer emotional support.

2. Seek Professional Guidance:

Speak with a reproductive endocrinologist or fertility specialist if possible. These professionals can provide insights into your specific situation and guide you through potential fertility treatments.

3. Join Support Groups:

Connect with others who are on similar journeys. Online and in-person support groups provide a space to share experiences, ask questions, and receive support from individuals who understand what you're going through.

4. Utilize Fertility Apps:

Explore fertility tracking apps that can help you monitor menstrual cycles, ovulation, and other key factors. These apps often provide valuable insights into your fertility patterns.

5. Fertility Education:

Arm yourself with knowledge about fertility. Understanding the basics of reproductive health, ovulation, and common fertility challenges empowers you to make informed decisions.

6. Online Resources:

Explore reputable online resources dedicated to fertility. Websites and forums, such as those provided by fertility clinics or health organizations, offer a wealth of information and can be valuable sources of support.

7. Fertility Counseling:

Consider seeking the support of a fertility counselor or therapist. They can provide emotional support, help you navigate the complexities of your feelings, and offer coping strategies.

8. Integrative Therapies:

Explore complementary and integrative therapies, such as acupuncture or mindfulness practices. These approaches may contribute to stress reduction and overall well-being.

9. Take Breaks When Needed:

Understand that taking breaks from actively trying to conceive is a valid and sometimes necessary choice. It allows you to recharge emotionally and mentally.

10. Financial Counseling:

If fertility treatments involve significant financial considerations, consider seeking financial counseling. Some clinics offer resources to help navigate the financial aspects of fertility treatments.

11. Maintain Open Communication:

Communicate openly with your partner about your feelings, fears, and hopes. Shared communication fosters a sense of unity and support.

12. Manage Stress Through Self-Care:

Prioritize self-care practices to manage stress. Whether it's taking walks, enjoying hobbies, or practicing relaxation techniques, finding ways to reduce stress is crucial.

13. Educational Workshops:

Attend workshops or seminars on fertility-related topics. These events often provide valuable insights, expert advice, and opportunities to connect with others.

14. Celebrate Milestones:

Celebrate milestones, whether big or small, along your fertility journey. Recognise and value your advancements.

15. Know Your Limits:

Recognize when you need to step back or seek professional help. Knowing your limits and seeking assistance when necessary is a sign of strength.

Practical Resources for Your Fertility Journey:

American Society for Reproductive Medicine (ASRM):

ASRM offers a wealth of information on reproductive health, including patient resources, fact sheets, and educational materials.

Resolve: The National Infertility Association:

Resolve provides support, advocacy, and resources for individuals and couples experiencing fertility challenges.

FertilityIQ:

FertilityIQ offers reviews and insights into fertility clinics, treatments, and medications, helping you make informed decisions.

My Fertility Navigator:

This online platform provides personalized guidance and resources for individuals navigating fertility treatments.

Fertility Preservation Network:

If fertility preservation is a consideration, the Fertility Preservation Network offers information and support for those facing medical treatments that may impact fertility.

Fertility Matters Canada:

This organization offers support and resources for Canadians dealing with fertility challenges.

Creating a Family:

Creating a Family provides a variety of resources, including podcasts, articles, and an online community for individuals on their fertility journey.

Books and Literature:

Explore literature on fertility and family-building. Books written by experts or individuals sharing their experiences can provide valuable insights.

Conclusion: Navigating Your Fertility Journey with Confidence

Your fertility journey is unique, and having the right support and resources can make a meaningful impact. By building a robust support network, accessing reliable resources, and prioritizing your well-being, you empower yourself to navigate the challenges and joys of this journey.

Here's to finding the support you need, gaining valuable insights, and approaching your fertility journey with confidence and resilience. May you discover the strength within you and the community around you as you move forward on this path.

CONCLUTION:

Embrace Your Journey to Wellness and Fertility

As we reach the final chapter of this book, it's time to reflect on the remarkable journey we've embarked on together. We've delved into the complexities of Polycystic Ovary Syndrome (PCOS), explored its effects on fertility, and learned how to manage it with a tailored IVF diet. We've discussed the importance of nutrient-rich foods, pre-IVF dietary recommendations, and the powerful role nutrition plays in preparing your body for IVF. Now, as we conclude, let's wrap it all up and leave you with a sense of fulfillment, inspiration, and a clear call to action.

The Essence of Your Journey

Your journey, like the pages of this book, is unique and personal. It's a path filled with hope, dreams, and challenges. At the heart of this journey is the unwavering belief that the power to create new life lies within you. And that belief is the essence of your journey.

Throughout this book, we've emphasized the significance of understanding PCOS, its impact on fertility, and the steps you can take to manage it. We've celebrated the vital role that nutrient-rich foods play in your quest for wellness and improved fertility. We've explored the dietary recommendations leading up to IVF, along with tips for nurturing your overall well-being. Now, as you prepare to close this chapter and continue your journey, let's revisit the core messages that will guide you forward.

Knowledge is Your North Star

Your journey began with knowledge, and knowledge remains your guiding light. You've gained a deeper understanding of PCOS and how it can affect your fertility. You've discovered that the right diet can be a potent tool in managing PCOS and optimizing your body for IVF. You now know the significance of nutrient-rich foods, balanced blood sugar, and personalized dietary recommendations. This knowledge is your strength, your foundation, and your compass.

Empowerment Through Nutrition

As you've explored the world of nutrition, you've unlocked a treasure trove of possibilities. You've come to appreciate the vibrant colors and flavors of fruits and vegetables, the nourishing power of lean proteins, and the role of healthy fats in hormonal balance. You've embraced the wisdom of supplements and the importance of hydration. And you've learned that stress management is an essential part of your wellness journey. All of these nutritional elements are like the tools in your toolbox, ready to support you every step of the way.

The Precious Moments Ahead

The road to wellness and improved fertility is not without its challenges, but it's also filled with the promise of joy, love, and new beginnings. The upcoming chapters of your life may include post-IVF considerations, the wonder of pregnancy, and the beauty of parenthood. These are moments of immense significance, and your journey has prepared you for them.

A Call to Action: Your Journey Continues

As we conclude this book, we want to leave you with a powerful call to action. Your journey doesn't end here; it's just beginning. The knowledge you've gained is a torch to light your way. The dietary recommendations are a roadmap to follow. The nutrient-rich foods are your daily companions, and the awareness of your own strength is your guiding star.

1. **Embrace Your Journey**: The path you're on is one of courage and determination. It's a journey where you carry the dreams of new life and the legacy of generations. Embrace it with open arms, for it's uniquely yours.

2. **Apply Your Knowledge**: Use the knowledge you've acquired. Make informed choices in your diet, in your lifestyle, and in your healthcare decisions. Your understanding of PCOS, fertility, and nutrition is a tool that empowers you.

3. **Seek Support**: You're not alone on this journey. Seek guidance and support from healthcare professionals, registered dietitians, and support groups. Share your experiences and listen to the stories of others who have walked similar paths.

4. **Stay Resilient**: Challenges may come, but you are resilient. Your ability to adapt, to learn, and to persevere is your greatest asset. The journey to wellness and improved fertility is a testament to your strength.

5. **Celebrate Your Victories**: Along the way, celebrate every victory, no matter how small. The steps you take, the changes you make, and the moments you savor are all part of the beautiful tapestry of your journey.

6. **Share Your Story**: Your journey is a story worth sharing. As you continue, consider sharing your experiences with others who may be on a similar path. Your story can be a beacon of hope and inspiration.

A Final Word: Your Journey to Wellness and Fertility

As you turn the final page of this book, remember that your journey is a testament to the strength of the human spirit, the power of knowledge, and the profound impact of nutrition on your path to wellness and improved fertility. Your story is still being written, and the chapters ahead are filled with moments of wonder, love, and new life.

With knowledge, determination, and a heart filled with hope, you have the power to shape your journey, to overcome obstacles, and to embrace the joy of parenthood. The road may be winding, but it's yours to travel, and your destination is filled with the promise of a brighter, happier future.

Your journey to wellness and fertility is a testament to the strength of the human spirit, the power of knowledge, and the profound impact of nutrition. You are the author of your story, and your journey is still being written. With every step, you are closer to the joy of parenthood. Your path may be filled with challenges, but it is also paved with the promise of love, new life, and the fulfillment of your dreams. The road ahead is yours to travel, and it's a journey filled with hope, courage, and boundless possibilities. Embrace it with an open heart, apply the knowledge you've gained, and know that your journey to wellness and fertility is a powerful story of resilience and strength. You are not alone on this path, and your story has the potential to inspire and uplift others. Celebrate every victory, no matter how small, and continue to share your experiences with those who may benefit from your guidance and support.

With every breath, every choice, and every moment, your journey to wellness and fertility is unfolding. May it be a journey of love, joy, and the fulfillment of your most cherished dreams. You are the author of your story, and the best chapters are yet to come.

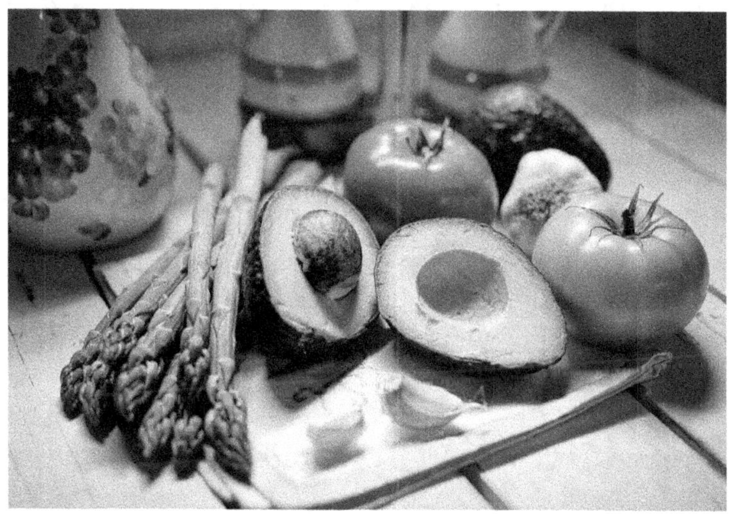

APPENDICES

Appendix A: Sample Meal Plans

Explore a variety of sample meal plans designed for individuals managing PCOS. These plans incorporate diverse and balanced recipes, offering inspiration for creating your customized PCOS-friendly meals.

Appendix B: Nutrient-Rich Recipes

Delve into a collection of nutrient-rich recipes tailored for PCOS and fertility support. From breakfast options to main courses and snacks, these recipes prioritize essential nutrients to enhance your well-being.

Appendix C: PCOS-Friendly Grocery List

Refer to a comprehensive grocery list specifically curated for individuals with PCOS. This resource simplifies your shopping experience, ensuring you have access to the key ingredients for maintaining a fertility-focused and balanced diet.

Appendix D: Fertility-Boosting Foods

Gain insights into a detailed list of fertility-boosting foods. This resource provides information on specific foods rich in antioxidants, vitamins, and minerals, supporting your fertility journey.

Appendix E: Tracking Your Menstrual Cycle

Utilize a menstrual cycle tracking template to monitor and understand your menstrual cycle. This appendix includes guidance on tracking ovulation, which can be valuable information for individuals trying to conceive.

Appendix F: Resources for Further Reading

Access a curated list of books, articles, and online resources for further exploration of PCOS, fertility, and related topics. This appendix serves as a gateway for readers interested in delving deeper into the subject matter.

Appendix G: Glossary of Terms

Refer to a glossary providing definitions of key terms related to PCOS, fertility, and nutritional concepts. This resource enhances readers' understanding by clarifying terminology used throughout the book.

Appendix H: Frequently Asked Questions (FAQs)

Find answers to commonly asked questions about PCOS, fertility, and dietary considerations. This appendix aims to address readers' queries and provide additional clarity on relevant topics.

Appendix I: Contact Information for Support Organizations

Access contact details for organizations specializing in PCOS support, fertility assistance, and related advocacy. This resource connects readers with valuable sources of assistance and community.

Note to Readers:
 These appendices are intended to complement the main content of the book, offering practical tools, additional information, and references for a more comprehensive understanding of PCOS, fertility, and the associated dietary considerations. Use these

appendices as valuable resources to support your journey towards improved well-being.